TABLE OF CONTE

MW00453541

Top 20 Test Taking Tips

1. Carefully follow all the test registration procedures
2. Know the test directions, duration, topics, question types, how many questions
3. Setup a flexible study schedule at least 3-4 weeks before test day
4. Study during the time of day you are most alert, relaxed, and stress free
5. Maximize your learning style; visual learner use visual study aids, auditory learner use auditory study aids
6. Focus on your weakest knowledge base
7. Find a study partner to review with and help clarify questions
8. Practice, practice, practice
9. Get a good night's sleep; don't try to cram the night before the test
10. Eat a well balanced meal
11. Know the exact physical location of the testing site; drive the route to the site prior to test day
12. Bring a set of ear plugs; the testing center could be noisy
13. Wear comfortable, loose fitting, layered clothing to the testing center; prepare for it to be either cold or hot during the test
14. Bring at least 2 current forms of ID to the testing center
15. Arrive to the test early; be prepared to wait and be patient
16. Eliminate the obviously wrong answer choices, then guess the first remaining choice
17. Pace yourself; don't rush, but keep working and move on if you get stuck
18. Maintain a positive attitude even if the test is going poorly
19. Keep your first answer unless you are positive it is wrong
20. Check your work, don't make a careless mistake

Anatomical Positions

Trendelengburg's Position: The body is laid flat on the back (supine position) with the feet higher than the head.

Shock Recovery Position: Feet and legs higher than the heart. It encourages blood flow back toward the heart and out of the peripheral tissues.

Flexion: Bending, most often ventrally to decrease the angle between two parts of the body; it is usually an action at an articulation or joint.

Extension: Straightening, or increasing the angle between two parts of the body; a stretching out or making the flexed part straight.

Abduction: A movement away from the midsagittal plane (midline); to adduct is to move medially and bring a part back to the mid-axis.

Circumduction: A circular movement at a ball and socket (shoulder or hip) joint, utilizing the movements of flexion, extension, abduction, and adduction.

Rotation: A movement of a part of the body around its long axis.

Supination: Refers only to the movement of the radius around the ulna. In supination the palm of the hand is oriented anteriorly; turning the palm dorsally puts it into pronation. The body on its back is in the supine position.

Pronation: Refers to the palm of the hand being oriented posteriorly. The body on its belly is the prone position.

Inversion: Refers only to the lower extremity, specifically the ankle joint. When the foot (plantar surface) is turned inward, so that the sole is pointing and directed toward the midline of the body and is parallel with the median plane, we speak of inversion. Its opposite is eversion.

Eversion: Refers to the foot (plantar surface) being turned outward so that the sole is pointing laterally.

Opposition: One of the most critical movements in humans; it allows us to have pulp-to-pulp opposition, which gives us the great dexterity of our hands. In this movement the thumb pad is brought to a finger pad. A median nerve injury negates this action.

Distal vs. *Proximal:* Self-explanatory

Prone position: Person lying on their stomach

Supine position: Person lying on their back

Nervous System

The nervous system is made of the central nervous system (CNS) and the peripheral nervous system (PNS). The central nervous system is made up of the brain and the spinal cord. The peripheral nervous system consists of cranial and spinal nerves that innervate organs, muscles and sensory systems. The brain controls: thought, reasoning, memory, sight, and judgment. The brain is made up of four lobes: frontal, parietal, temporal, and occipital. The spinal cord is a made up of neural tracts that conduct information to and from the brain.

Cranial nerves in the peripheral nervous system connect the brain to the head, neck and trunk. Peripheral nerves allow control of muscle groups in the upper and lower extremities and sensory stimulation. The peripheral nerves are spinal nerves that branch off the spinal cord going toward organs, and muscles.

The autonomic nervous system controls reflexive functions of the brain. Including "fight or flight" response and maintaining homeostasis. Homeostasis is a state of equilibrium within tissues. The autonomic nervous system uses neurotransmitters to help conduct nerve signals and turn on/off various cell groups.

Nervous tissue is composed of neurons, which are the functional unit of the nervous system. A neuron includes a cell body, and organelles usually found in cells. Dendrites provide receptive information to the neuron and a single axon carries the information away.

Key terms

Synapse: Junction between two neurons

Action potential: Threshold at which neurons fire

The brain

Frontal lobe: Controls emotions, judgments, controls motor aspects of speech, primary motor cortex for voluntary muscle activation

Parietal lobe: Receives fibers with sensory information about touch, proprioception, temperature, and pain from the other side of the body

Temporal lobe: Responsible for auditory information, and language comprehension

Occipital lobe: Center for visual information

Cerebellum: Coordination of muscle function

Brainstem (midbrain, pons, and medulla) – Respiratory and cardiac center, nerve pathways to the brain

Diencephalon: (thalamus, subthalamus, and hypothalamus)

Thalamus: Integrate and relay sensory information from the face, retina, cochlea, and taste receptors. Interprets sensation of touch, pain and temperature

Hypothalamus: Controls the autonomic nervous system and the neuroendocrine systems, maintains body homeostasis, helps regulate body temperature, helps regulate appetite control, thirst center, sleeping cycle, and control of hormone secretion.

Glasgow Coma Scale

+Eye Opening

+Best Motor Response

+Best Verbal Response

Total (3-15 Score Range) A score of 1 in each category indicates no performance of skill.

Autonomic nervous system

Sympathetic (Fight or Flight): Dilated pupils, elevates heart rate and respiratory rate, sweating, epinephrine and norepinephrine secreted, increased blood pressure, and constriction of skin and abdominal arterioles.

Parasympathetic: Constricted pupils, lowers heart rate and respiratory rate, increased peristalsis, acetylcholine secreted, decreases blood pressure, and relaxation of skin and abdominal arterioles.

Cranial nerves

I	Olfactory:	Smell
II	Optic:	Vision acuity
III	Oculomotor:	Eye function
IV	Trochlear:	Eye function
V	Trigeminal:	Sensory of the face, chewing
VI	Abducens:	Eye function
VII	Facial:	Facial expression, wrinkle forehead, taste anterior tongue
VIII	Vestibulocochlear:	Auditory acuity, balance and postural responses
IX	Glossopharyngeal:	Taste on posterior 33% of the scale
X	Vagus:	Cardiac, respiratory reflexes
XI	Spinal Accessory:	Strength of trapezius and Sternocleidomastoid muscles
XII	Hypoglossal:	Motor function of the tongue

Key terms

Apraxia: Inability to perform purposeful movements

Agnosia: Inability to recognize familiar objects by the various senses

Spasticity: Increased tone, hyperactive reflexes, clonus, +Babinski

Ataxia: General term used to describe uncoordinated movement; may influence gait, posture, and patterns of movements

Chorea: Involuntary, rapid, irregular, jerky movements, clinical feature of Huntington disease

Flaccidity: Absent tone

Hypotonia: Decreased tone

Expressive Aphasia: Inability to speak or difficulty speaking

Receptive Aphasia: Inability to understand verbal speech, inability to receive information

Stroke Factors and Aneurysm Precautions

Stroke factors include: Diabetes, atherosclerosis, hypertension, cardiac disease, and transient ischemic attacks

Aneurysm precautions include: Avoid rectal temperatures, limit visitors, avoid Valsalva's maneuver, and the head of bed should be between 30-45 degrees.

Miscellaneious Brain Diseases

Valsalva's maneuver: Occurs when attempting to forcibly exhale with the glottis, mouth and nose closed. It causes an increase in intrathoracic pressure with an accompanying collapse of the vein of the chest wall. The following may result: Slowing of the pulse, decreased return of blood to the heart, and increased intrathoracic pressure

Horner's Syndrome: Sympathetic innervation to the face is interrupted by a lesion in the brain stem resulting in pupillary constriction, dry and red face with no sweat.

Autonomic Dysreflexia: Caused by a lesion in the high thoracic or cervical cord. Severe hypertension, sweating and headaches noted. May occur with a blockage in a urine catheter.

Parkinson's Disease: A degenerative disease with primary involvement of the basal ganglia; characterized by the following: Bradykinesia, resting tremor and emotional lability.

Multiple Sclerosis: Progressive demyelinating disease of the central nervous system affecting mostly young adults. Causes are unknown, most likely viral. Symptoms include: Demyelinating lesions limit neural transmission, mild to moderate impaired cognition common, sensory deficits, bowel and bladder deficits, and spasticity is common.

Myasthenia gravis: Neuromuscular disease characterized by fatigue of skeletal muscles and muscular weakness.

Guillain-Barre' Syndrome: Polyneuropathy with progressive muscular weakness

Amyotrophic lateral sclerosis (Lou Gehrig's disease) – degenerative disease affecting upper and lower motor neurons

Post-polio Syndrome- slowly progressive muscle weakness that occurs in patients with a history of acute poliomyelitis, after a stable period

Meningitis: Inflammation of the meninges of the spinal cord and brain caused by bacteria.

APGAR score: (Appearance, Pulse, Grimace, Activity, Respiration) (0-2) each category: Color, heart rate, reflex irritability, muscle tone, and respiratory effort.

Seizures

Epilepsy: Recurrent seizures due to excessive and sudden discharge of cerebral cortical neurons.

Tonic-clonic (Grand Mal): Patient is confused and drowsy about the seizures, 2-5 min generally.

Absence seizures (Petit Mal): Brief, no convulsive contractions, may be up to 100X day

Simple Seizures: No loss of consciousness

Complex Seizures: Brief loss of consciousness with psychomotor changes
***Key Point*- When a patient has a seizure during most interventions, do not use a tongue blade and allow free movement in a safe environment

Respiratory Review

The respiratory stem includes the nose, nasal cavity, sinuses, pharynx, larynx, trachea, bronchial tree, and lungs. Air enters the nose, travels through the nasal cavity where the air is warmed. The air goes through the pharynx, which functions as a common duct for air and food. Then the larynx, which is at the top of the trachea and holds the vocal cords and allows passage of air. The trachea divides into the right and left bronchi on the way into the bronchial tree and the lungs.

The right lung has three lobes and the left lung has two lobes. Gas exchange occurs between the air and the blood within the alveoli, which are tiny air sacs. Diffusion is the mechanism by which oxygen and carbon dioxide are exchanged.

Breathing is controlled by the medulla oblongata and pons. Inspiration is controlled by changes in the thoracic cavity. Air fills the lung because of atmospheric pressure pushing air in. Expansion of the lungs is aided by surface tension, which holds pleural membranes together. In addition, the diaphragm, which is located just below the lungs, and stimulated by phrenic nerve, acts as a suction pump to encourage inspiration. Expiration comes from the recoil of tissues and the surface tension of the alveoli.

Aerobic respiration occurs in the presence of oxygen and mostly takes place in the mitochondria of a cell. Anaerobic respiration occurs in the absence of oxygen and takes place in the cytoplasm of a cell. Both of these mechanisms occur in cellular respiration in humans. With anaerobic respiration glucose is broken down and produces less ATP when compared to aerobic respiration.

Respiratory terms

Tidal volume: Amount of air that is inhaled and exhaled during normal resting ventilation

Residual volume: The amount of air remaining in the lungs following a maximal expiration

ERV (Expiratory reserve volume): The volume of air that can be forcefully expelled following a normal expiration

IRV (Inspiratory reserve volume): The volume of air that can be forcefully breathed in following a normal inspiration

FVC (Forced vital capacity): IRV +TV +ERV

FEV1 (Forced expiratory volume): The volume of air that can be forcefully expelled in one second following a full inspiration.

Total lung capacity: Sum of the residual volume and the vital capacity

Functional residual capacity: The volume of air remaining in the lungs following a normal expiration or ERV + RV

Metabolic Equivalent (MET): A rating of energy expenditure for a given activity based on oxygen consumption. One MET equals 3.5 ml of oxygen used per kilogram of body weight per minute.

CO = SV x HR

(Cardiac Output) = (Stroke Volume) x (Heart Rate)

$$EF = \frac{SV}{EDV} * 100\%$$

$$(\text{Ejection fraction}) = \frac{(\text{Stroke volume})}{(\text{End diastolic volume})}$$

Breath sounds

Friction rub: Caused by the rubbing of pleural surfaces against one another, usually as the result of inflammation processes.

Rales (crackles): Adventitious breath sounds associated with pathology. Rales could be the result of air bubbles in secretions or movement of fibrotic tissue during breathing. Basilar rales are often accompanied with left ventricular congestive heart failure. (Atelectasis, fibrosis, and pulmonary edema) are related to the opening of previously closed small airways and alveoli.

Rhonchi: Continuous low pitched, sonorous breath sounds that are most prominent during expiration and could be a result of air passing through airways narrowed by inflammation, bronchospasm or secretions. Heard during expiration

Stridor: Continuous adventitious sound of inspiration associated with upper airway obstruction

Wheezes: Continuous breath sounds that are high-pitched, and musical often associated with asthma, COPD, and foreign body aspiration

Know This Chart Backwards and Forwards

Acid/Base Balance	pH	Causes
Respiratory Alkalosis	Up	Alveolar hyperventilation
Respiratory Acidosis	Down	Alveolar hypoventilation
Metabolic Alkalosis	Up	(Steroids, adrenal disease)
Metabolic Acidosis	Down	(Diabetic, prolonged diarrhea)

Key Point : Hyperventilation may result in Respiratory Alkalosis

Normative Values for Infants/Adults

Term	Infant	Adult
HR	120bpm	60-100bpm
BP	75/50 mmHg	120/80 mmHg
RR	40	12-18
pH	7.26-7.41	7.35-7.45
Tidal Volume	20 ml	500 ml

COPD-Chronic Bronchitis/Emphysema-abnormal expiratory flow rates.

Chronic Bronchitis, Emphysema, and Tuberculosis

Chronic Bronchitis signs and symptoms: Smoking history, decreased expiratory flow rates, crackles and wheezes, and hypoxemia.

Emphysema signs and symptoms: Barrel chest, dyspnea, cyanosis, clubbing, and accessory muscles of ventilation.

Tuberculosis: Infectious respiratory process caused by tubercle bacilli.

Terminology

Orthopnea: Difficulty breathing in positions other than upright sitting and standing

Orthostatic hypotension: Decrease in blood pressure upon assuming an erectposture. This is normal, but may be excessive resulting in fainting.

Atelectasis: Alveolar collapse involving part or all of the lung due to the complete absorption of gas or the inability of the alveoli to expand

Apnea: Absence of respirations, usually temporary in duration

Bradycardia: Abnormally slow (low) pulse rate; below approximately 50 beats per minute.

Cor pulmonale: Right ventricular enlargement from a primary pulmonary cause

Cheyne-Strokes: Respiration-breathing pattern characterized by a gradual increase in rate and depth followed by a gradual decrease; periods of apnea occur between cycles.

Tachycardia: Abnormally rapid (high) pulse rate; over approximately 100 beats per minute.

Beta-adrenergic blocking agents (beta-blockers): Propranolol, Metoprolol, nadolol, Atenolol, Timolol

Calcium channel blocking agent: Verapamil, Nifedipine, Diltiazem – A substance that inhibits the flow of calcium ions across membranes in smooth muscle. These drugs cause vasodilation and relieve angina pain and coronary artery spasm.

Ejection fraction: Difference between left ventricular end diastolic volume and left ventricular end systolic volume.

Digitalis: A drug that strengthens the contraction of the heart muscle, slows the rate of contraction of the heart, and promotes the elimination of fluid from body tissues.

Antiarrhythmics: Lidocaine, Quinidine, Procainamide, Disopyramide, Phenytoin (Dilantin) – Agents used to treat cardiac arrhythmias.

Catecholamines: Circulating compounds (epinephrine and norepinephrine) that are secreted by the sympathetic nervous system and the adrenal medulla; they act to increase cardiac rate, contractility, automaticity, and excitability.

Respiratory Conditions

Pulmonary Valve Stenosis

Causes: Congenital, endocarditis, rheumatic fever

Symptoms: Fainting, SOB, palpitations, cyanosis, poor weight gain

Tests: Cardiac catheterization, ECG, chest-xray, echocardiogram

Treatment: Prostaglandins, dieuretics, anti-arrhythmics, blood thinners, valvuloplasty

ARDS

Low oxygen levels caused by a build up of fluid in the lungs and inflammation of lung tissue.

Causes: Trauma, chemical inhalation, pneumonia, septic shock

Symptoms: Low BP, rapid breathing, SOB

Tests: ABG, CBC, cultures

Treatment: Echocardiogram, auscultation, cyanosis, chest X-ray, mechanical ventilation, treat the underlying condition

Monitor the Patient for: Pulmonary fibrosis, multiple system organ failure, ventilator associated pneumonia, acidosis, respiratory failure

Respiratory Acidosis

Build-up of Carbon Dioxide in the lungs that causes acid-base imbalances and the body becomes acidic.

Causes: COPD, airway obstruction, hypoventilation syndrome, *severe scoliosis, severe asthma*

Symptoms: Chronic cough, wheezing, SOB, confusion, fatigue

Tests: CAT scan, ABG, pulmonary function test

Treatment: Mechanical ventilation, bronchodilators

Respiratory Alkalosis

CO2 levels are reduced and pH is high.

Causes: Anxiety, fever, hyperventilation

Symptoms: Dizziness, numbness

Tests: ABG, chest x-ray, pulmonary function test

Treatment: Paper bag technique, increase carbon dioxide levels

RSV (Respiratory synctial virus)

Spread by contact, virus can survive for various time periods on different surfaces.

Symptoms: Fever, SOB, cyanosis, wheezing, nasal congestion, croupy cough

Tests: ABG, chest x-ray

Treatment: Ribvirin, ventilator in severe cases, IV fluids, bronchodilators

Monitor the patient for: Pneumonia, respiratory failure, otitis media

Hyperventilation, apnea and lung surgery

Causes of hyperventilation: COPD, panic attacks, stress, ketoacidosis, aspirin overdose, anxiety

Apnea: No spontaneous breathing

Causes: Obstructive sleep apnea, seizures, cardiac arrhythmias, brain injury, nervous system dysfunction, drug overdose, prematurity, bronchospasm, encephalitis, choking

Lung surgery causes: Cancer, lung abscesses, atelectasis, emphysema, pneumothorax, tumors, bronchiectasis

Pneumonia

Viruses are the primary cause in young children; bacteria the primary cause in adults.

Bacteria: Streptococcus pneumoniae, Mycoplasma pneumoniae (pneumococcus)

Types of pneumonia: Viral pneumonia, walking pneumonia, legionella pneumonia, CMV pneumonia, Aspiration pneumonia, Atypical pneumonia

Symptoms: Fever, headache, ribvirin, SOB, cough, chest pain

Tests: Chest x-ray, pulmonary perfusion scan, CBC, cultures of sputum, presence of crackles

Treatment: Antibiotics if caused by a bacterial infection, respiratory treatments, steroids, IV fluids, vaccine treatments

Alveolar proteinosis

A build-up of a phospholipid in the lungs were carbon dioxide and oxygen are transferred.

Causes: May be associated with infection, genetic disorder 30-50 yrs. Old

Symptoms: Weight loss, fatigue, cough, fever, SOB

Tests: Chest x-ray, presence of crackles, CT scan, bronchoscopy, ABG – low 02 levels, pulmonary function tests

Treatment: Lung transplantation, special lavage of the lungs

Pulmonary actinomycosis

Bacteria infection of the lungs caused by (propionibacteria or actinomyces)

Causes: Microorganisms

Symptoms: Pleural effusions, facial lesions, chest pain, cough, weight loss, fever

Tests: CBC, lung biopsy, thoracentesis, CT scan, bronchoscopy

Monitor patient for: Emphysema, meningitis, osteomyelitis

Pulmonary hypertension

Causes: Elevated BP in the lung arteries, may be genetically linked, more predomant in women

Symptoms: Fainting, fatigue, chest pain, SOB with activity, LE edema, weakness

Tests: Pulmonary arteriogram, chest x-ray, ECG, pulmonary function tests, CT scan, cardiac catheterization

Treatment: Manage symptoms, diuretics, calcium channel blockers, heart or lung transploant if necessary

Pulmonary arteriovenous fistulas

A congenital defect where lung arteries and veins form improperly, and a fistula is formed creating poor oxygenation of blood.

Symptoms: SOB with activity, presence of a murmur, cyanosis, clubbing, paradoxical embolism

Tests: CT Scan, pulmonary arteriogram, low O2 saturation levels, elevated RBC's

Treatment: Surgery, embolization

Pulmonary aspergilloma

Fungal infection of the lung cavities causing abscesses.

Cause: Fungus *Aspergillus*

Symptoms: Wheezing, SOB, chest pain, fever, cough

Tests: CT scan, sputum culture, serum precipitans, chest x-ray, bronchoscopy

Treatment: Surgery, antifungalmedications

Pulmonary edema

Most commonly caused by Heart Failure, but may be due to lung disorders.

Symptoms: Restless behavior, anxiety, wheezing, poor speech, SOB, sweating, pale skin, drowning sensation

Tests: Murmurs may be present, echocardiogram, presence of crackles, low O2 saturation levels

Treatment: Diuretics, oxygen, treat the underlying cause

Idiopathic pulmonary fibrosis

Thickening of lung tissue in the lower aspects of the lungs

Causes: Response to an inflammatory agent, , found in people ages 50-70, linked to smoking

Symptoms: Cough, SOB, chest pain, cyanosis, clubbing, cyanosis

Tests: Pulmonary function tests, lung biopsy, rule out other connective tissue diseases, CT scan, chest X-ray

Monitor the patient for: Polycythemia

Treatment: Lung transplantation, corticosteroids, anti-inflammatory drug, pulmonary Htn, respiratory failure, cor pulmonarle

Pulmonary emboli

Blood clot of the pulmonary vessels or blockage due to fat droplets, tumors or parasites.

Causes: DVT- most common

Symptoms: SOB (rapid onset), chest pain, decreased BP, skin color changes, LE and pelvic pain, sweating, dizziness, anxiety, tachycardia, labored breathing, cough

Tests: Doppler US, chest x-ray, pulmonary angiogram, pulmonary perfusion test, plethysmography, ABG, check O2 saturation

Treatment: Placement of an IVC filter, administer oxygen, surgery, thrombolytic therapy if clot detected

Monitor the patient for: Shock, pulmonary hypertension, hemorrhage, palipitations, heart failure

Tuberculosis

Infection caused by *Mycobaterium tuberculosis.*

Causes: Due to airborne exposure

Symptoms: Fever, chest pain, SOB, weight loss, fatigue, wheezing, phlegm production, presence of crackles

Tests: Thoracentesis, sputum cultures, TB skin test, chest X-ray, bronchoscopy

Treatment: Generally about 6 months, Rifampin, Pyrazinamide, Isoniazid

Cytomegalovirus

Can cause lung infections and is a herpes-type virus.

Causes: More common in immunocompromised patients; Often associated with organ transplantation

Symptoms: Fever, SOB, fatigue, loss of appetite, cough, joint pain

Tests: CMV serology tests, ABG, bood cultures, bronchoscopy

Treatment: Antiviral medications, oxygen therapy

Monitor the patient for: Kidney dysfunction, infection, decreased WBC levels, relapses

Viral pneumonia

Inflammation of the lungs caused by viral infection

Causes: Rhinovirus, herpes simplex virus, influenza, adenovirus, hantavirus, CMV, RSV

Symptoms: Fatigue, sore throats, nausea, joint pain, headaches, muscular pain, cough, SOB

Tests: Bronchoscopy, open lung biopsy, sputum cultures, viral blood tests

Treatment: Antiviral medications, IV fluids

Monitor the patient for: Liver failure, heart failure, respiratory failure

Pneumothorax

A build-up of a gas in the pleural cavities.

Types: Traumatic pneumothorax, tension pneumothorax, spontaneous pneumothorax, secondary spontaneous pneumothorax

Symptoms: SOB, tachycardia, hypotension, anxiety, cyanosis, chest pain-sharp, fatigue

Tests: ABG and chest x-ray, poor breath sounds

Treatment: Chest tube insertion, administration of oxygen

Circulatory System

Functions

The circulatory system serves to:

- Conduct nutrients and oxygen to the tissues;

- Remove waste materials by transporting nitrogenous compounds to the kidneys and carbon dioxide to the lungs;

- Transport chemical messengers (hormones) to target organs and modulate and integrate the internal milieu of the body;

- Transport agents which serve the body in allergic, immune, and infectious responses;

- Initiate clotting and thereby prevent blood loss;

- Maintain body temperature;

- Produce, carry and contain blood;

- Transfer body reserves, specifically mineral salts, to areas of need.

General Components and Structure

The circulatory system consists of the heart, blood vessels, blood and lymphatics. It is a network of tubular structures through which blood travels to and from all the parts of the body. In vertebrates this is a completely closed circuit system, as William Harvey (1628) once demonstrated. The heart is a modified, specialized, powerful pumping blood vessel. Arteries, eventually becoming arterioles, conduct blood to capillaries (essentially endothelial tubes), and venules, eventually becoming veins, return blood from the capillary bed to the heart.

Course of Circulation

Arterial system: Blood is delivered by the pulmonary veins (two from each lung) to the left atrium, passes through the bicuspid (mitral) valve into the left ventricle and then is pumped into the ascending aorta; backflow here is prevented by the aortic semilunar valves. The aortic arch toward the right side gives rise to the brachiocephalic (innominate) artery which divides into the right subclavian and right common carotid arteries. Next, arising from the arch is the common carotid artery, then the left subclavian artery.

The subclavians supply the upper limbs. As the subclavian arteries leave the axilla (armpit) and enter the arm (brachium), they are called brachial arteries. Below the elbow these main trunk lines divide into ulnar and radial arteries, which supply the forearm and eventually form a set of arterial arches in the hand which give rise to common and proper digital arteries. The descending (dorsal) aorta continues along the posterior aspect of the thorax giving rise to the segmental intercostals arteries. After passage "through" (behind) the diaphragm it is called the abdominal aorta.

At the pelvic rim the abdominal aorta divides into the right and left common iliac arteries. These divide into the internal iliacs, which supply the pelvic organs, and the external iliacs, which supply the lower limb.

Venous system: Veins are frequently multiple and variations are common. They return blood originating in the capillaries of peripheral and distal body parts to the heart.

Hepatic Portal System: Blood draining the alimentary tract (intestines), pancreas, spleen and gall bladder does not return directly to the systemic circulation, but is relayed by the hepatic portal system of veins to and through the liver. In the liver, absorbed foodstuffs and wastes are processed. After processing, the liver returns the blood via hepatic veins to the inferior vena cava and from there to the heart.

Pulmonary Circuit: Blood is oxygenated and depleted of metabolic products such as carbon dioxide in the lungs.

Lymphatic Drainage: A network of lymphatic capillaries permeates the body tissues. Lymph is a fluid similar in composition to blood plasma, and tissue fluids not reabsorbed into blood capillaries are transported via the lymphatic system eventually to join the venous system at the junction of the left internal jugular and subclavian veins.

The heart

The heart is a highly specialized blood vessel which pumps 72 times per minute and propels about 4,000 gallons (about 15,000 liters) of blood daily to the tissues. It is composed of:

> Endocardium (lining coat; epithelium)
> Myocardium (middle coat; cardiac muscle)
> Epicardium (external coat or visceral layer of pericardium; epithelium and mostly connective tissue)
> Impulse conducting system

Cardiac Nerves

Modification of the intrinsic rhythmicity of the heart muscle is produced by cardiac nerves of the sympathetic and parasympathetic nervous system. Stimulation of the sympathetic system increases the rate and force of the heartbeat and dilates the coronary arteries. Stimulation of the parasympathetic (vagus nerve) reduces the rate and force of the heartbeat and constricts the coronary circulation. Visceral afferent (sensory) fibers from the heart end almost wholly in the first four segments of the thoracic spinal cord.

Cardiac Cycle

Alternating contraction and relaxation is repeated about 75 times per minute; the duration of one cycle is about 0.8 second. Three phases succeed one another during the cycle:

- atrial systole: 0.1 second,
- ventricular systole: 0.3 second,
- diastole: 0.4 second

The actual period of rest for each chamber is 0.7 second for the atria and 0.5 second for the ventricles, so in spite of its activity, the heart is at rest longer than at work.

Blood

Blood is composed of cells (corpuscles) and a liquid intercellular ground substance called plasma. The average blood volume is 5 or 6 liters (7% of body weight). Plasma constitutes about 55% of blood volume, cellular elements about 45%.

Plasma

Over 90% of plasma is water; the balance is made up of plasma proteins and dissolved electrolytes, hormones, antibodies, nutrients, and waste products. Plasma is isotonic (0.85% sodium chloride). Plasma plays a vital role in respiration, circulation, coagulation, temperature regulation, buffer activities and overall fluid balance.

Cardiovascular conditions

<u>Shock</u>

Cardiogenic Shock: Heart is unable to meet the demands of the body. This can be caused by conduction system failure or heart muscle dysfunction.

Symptoms of Shock: Rapid breathing, rapid pulse, anxiety, nervousness, thready pulse, mottled skin color, profuse sweating, poor capillary refill

Tests: Nuclear scans, electrocardiogram, echocardiogram, electrocardiogram, ABG, chem-7, chem-20, electrolytes, cardiac enzymes

Treatment: Amrinone, norepinephrine, dobutamine, IV fluids, PTCA, extreme cases-pacemaker, IABP

Hypovolemic shock: Poor blood volume prevents the heart from pumping enough blood to the body.

Causes: Trauma, diarrhea, burns, GI Bleeding

Cardiogenic shock: Enough blood is available; however the heart is unable to move the blood in an effective manner.

Symptoms: Anxiety, weakness, sweating, rapid pulse, confusion, clammy skin

Tests: CBC, echocardiogram, CT scan, endoscopy with GI bleeding, Swan-Ganz catheterization

Treatment: Increase fluids via IV; avoid hypothermia, epinephrine, norepinephrine, dobutamine, and dopamine

<u>Aortic insufficiency</u>

Heart valve disease that prevents the aortic valve from closing completely; backflow of blood into the left ventricle.

Causes: Rheumatic fever, congenital abnormalities, endocarditis, Marfan's syndrome, Ankylosing spondylitis, Reiter's syndrome

Symptoms: Fainting, weakness, bounding pulse, SOB, fatigue

Tests: Palpation, increased pulse pressure and diastolic pressure, pulmonary edema present, auscultation, left heart chatereterization, aortica angiography, Dopper US, echocardiogram

Treatment: Digoxin, dieuretics, surgical aorta valve repair

Monitor patient for: PE, left sided heart failure, endocarditis

Aortic aneurysm

Expansion of the blood vessel wall often identified in the thoracic region.

Causes: Htn, Marfan's syndrome, syphilis, atherosclerosis (most common), trauma

Symptoms: Possible back pain may be the only indicator

Tests: Aortogram, chest CT, chest x-ray

Treatment: Varies depending on location, stent, circulatory arrest, surgery

Monitor patient for: Bleeding, stroke, graft infection, irregular heartbeats, and heart attack

Myocarditis

Inflammation of the heart muscle.

Causes: Bacterial or viral infections, polio, adenovirus, coxsackie virus

Symptoms: Leg edema, SOB, viral symptoms, joint pain, syncope, heart attack (pain), fever, unable to lie flat, irregular heart beats

Tests: Chest x-ray, echocardiogram, ECG, *WBC and RBC count, blood cultures*

Treatment: Diuretics, pacemaker, antibiotics, steroids

Monitor the patient for: Pericarditis and cardiomyopathy

Heart valve infection

Endocarditis (inflammation), probable valvular heart disease; can be caused by fungi or bacteria.

Symptoms: Weakness, fever, murmur, SOB, night sweats, Janeway lesions, joint pain

Tests: CBC, ESR, ECG, blood cultures, enlarged speen, presence of splinter, hemorrhages

Treatment: IV antibiotics, surgery may be indicated

Monitor the patient for: Jaundice, arrhythmias, CHF, glomerulonephritis, emboli

Pericarditis

Inflammation of the pericardium.

Causes: Viral (Coxsackie), adenovirus, influenza, rubella viruses, bacterial (various microorganisms), fungi, often associated with TB, kidney failure, AIDS, and autoimmune disorders, surgery

Symptoms: Dry cough, pleuritis, fever, anxiety, crackles, pleural effusion, LE swelling, chest pain, unable to lie down flat

Tests: Auscultation, MRI scan, CT scan, Echocardiogram (key test), ESR, chest x-ray, blood cultures, CBC

Treatment: NSAIDS, pericardiocentesis, analgesics, pericardiectomy

Monitor the patient for: Constrictive pericarditis, A fib., upraventricular tachycardia (SVT)

Arrhythmias

Irregular heart beats and rhythms disorder

Types: Bradycardia, tachycardia, Ventricular fibrillation, Ectopic heart beat, ventricular tachycardia, Wolff-Parkinson-white syndrome, atrial fib., sick sinus syndrome, sinus tachycardia, sinus bradycardia

Symptoms: SOB, fainting, palpitations, dizziness, chest pain, irregular pulse

Tests: Coronary angiography, ECG, echocardiogram, holter monitor

Treatment: Defibrillation, pacemaker, medications

Monitor the patient for: Heart failure, stroke, heart attack, ischemia

Arteriosclerosis

Hardening of the arteries

Causes: Smoking, Htn, kidney disease, CAD, stroke

Symptoms: Claudication pain, cold feet, muscle acheness and pain in the legs, hair loss on the legs, numbness in the extremities, weak distal pulse

Tests: Doppler US, angiography, IVSU, MRI test, poor ABI (Ankle brachial index) reading

Treatment: Analgesics, vasodilation medications, surgery if severe, Balloon surgery, stent placement

Monitor the patient for: Arterial emboli, ulcers, impotence, gas gangreene, infection of the lower extremities

Cardiomyopathy

Poor hear pumping and weakness of the myocardium.

Causes: Htn, heart attacks, viral infections

Types:

- Alcoholic cardiomyopathy: Due to alcohol consumption
- Dilated cardiomyopathy: Left ventricle enlargement
- Hypertrophic cardiomyopathy: Abnormal growth left ventricle
- Ischemic cardiomyopathy: Weakness of the myocardium due to heart attacks.
- Peripartum cardiomyopathy: Found in late pregnancy
- Restrictive cardiomyopathy: Limited filling of the heart due to inability to relax heart tissue.

Symptoms: Chest pain, SOB, fatigue, ascites, LE swelling, fainting, poor appetite Htn, palpitations

Tests: ECG, CBC, Isoenzyme tests, Coronary Angigraphy, chest x-ray, MRI, auscultation

Treatment: Ace inhibitors, dieuretics, blood thinners, Left Ventricular Assist Device (LVAD), digoxin, vasodilators

Heart Sounds:

S1 – Tricuspid and mitral valve close

S2 – Pulmonary and aortic valve close

S3 – Ventricular filling complete

S4 – Elevated atrial pressure (atrial kick)

Wave Review:

ST segment: Ventricles depolarized

P wave: Atrial depolarization

PR segment: AV node conduction

QRS complex: Ventricular depolarization

U wave: Hypokalemia creates a U wave

T wave: Ventricular repolarization

Wave Review Indepth:

P WAVE: Small upward wave; indicates atrial depolarization

QRS COMPLEX: Initial downward deflection followed by large upright wave followed by small downward wave; represents ventricular depolarization; masks atrial repolarization; enlarged R portion - enlarged ventricles; enlarged Q portion - probable heart attack.

T WAVE: Dome shaped wave; indicates ventricular repolarization; flat when insufficient oxygen; elevated with increased K levels

P - R INTERVAL: Interval from beginning of P wave to R wave; represents conduction time from initial atrial excitation to initial ventricular excitation; good diagnostic tool; normally < 0.2sec.

S-T SEGMENT: Time from end of S to beginning to T wave; represents time between end of spreading impulse through ventricles and ventricular repolarization; elevated with heart attack; depressed when insufficient oxygen.

Q-T INTERVAL: Time for singular depolarization and repolarization of the ventricles. Conduction problems, myocardial damage or congenital heart defects can prolong this.

Arrhythmias review

<u>Supraventricular Tachyarrhythmias</u>

Atrial fibrillation: Abnormal QRS rhythm and poor P wave appearance. (>300bpm)

Sinus Tachycardia: Elevated ventricular rhythum/rate.

Paroxysmal atrial tachycardia: Abnormal P wave, Normal QRS complex

Atrial flutter: Irregular P Wave development. (250-350 bpm)

Paroxysmal supraventricular tachycardia: Elevated bpm (160-250)

Multifocal atrial tachycardia: Various P wave appearances. (bpm >105)

<u>Ventricular Tachyarrhythmias</u>

Ventricular Tachycardia: Presence of 3 or greater PVC's (150-200bpm), possible abrupt onset. Possibly due to an ischemic ventricle. No P waves present.

Premature Ventricular Contraction (PVC): In many cases no P wave followed by a large QRS complex that is premature, followed by a compensatory pause.

Ventricular fibrillation: Completely abnormal ventricular rate and rhythum requiring emergency innervention. No effective cardiac output.

<u>Bradyarrhythmias</u>

AV block (primary, secondary (I,II) Tertiary

Primary: >.02 PR interval

Secondary (Mobitz I): PR interval Increase

Secondary (Mobitz II): PR interval (no change)

Tertiary: Most severe, No signal between ventricles and atria noted on ECG. Probable use of Atrophine indicated. Pacemaker required.

Right Bundle Branch Block (RBBB)/Left Bundle Branch Block (LBBB)

Sinus Bradycardia – V<60 bpm, with presence of a standard P wave.

Cardiac failure review

Right Sided Heart Failure

Symptoms of right sided heart failure: Right upper quadrant pain, right ventricular heave, tricuspid murmur, weight gain, nausea, elevated right atrial pressure, elevated central venous pressure, peripheral edema, ascites, anorexia, hepatomegaly

Left Sided Heart Failure

Symptoms of left sided heart failure: Left ventricular heave, confusion, paroxysmal noturnal dyspnea, DOE, fatigue, S3 gallop, crackles, tachycardia, cough, mitral murmur, diaphoresis, orthopnea

ECG Changes

With MI: T Wave inversion, ST Segment Elevation, abnormal Q waves

With Digitalis: Inverts T wave, QT segment shorter, depresses ST segment

With Quinidine: Inverts T wave, QT segment longer, QRS segment longer

With Potassium:

- Hyperkalemia: Lowers P wave, Increases width of QRS complex
- Hypokalemia: Lowers T wave, causes a U wave

With Calcium:

- Hypercalcemia: Makes a longer QRS segment
- Hypocalcemia: Increases time of QT interval

Endocrine Review

Hypothyroidism

Poor production of thyroid hormone:

Primary – Thyroid cannot meet the demands of the pituitary gland.

Secondary – No stimulation of the thyroid by the pituitary gland.

Causes: Surgical thyroid removal, irradiation, congenital defects, Hashimoto's thyroiditis (key)

Symptoms: Constipation, weight gain, weakness, fatigue, poor taste, hoarse vocal sounds, joint pain, muscle weakness, poor speech, color changes, depression

Tests: Decreased BP and HR; chest X-ray; elevated liver enzymes, prolactin, and cholesterol; decreased T4 levels and serum sodium levels; presence of anemia; low temperature; and poor reflexes

Treatment: Increase thyroid hormone levels, Levothyroxine

Monitor the patient for: Hyperthyroidism symptoms following treatment, heart disease, miscarriage, Myxedema coma if untreated

Hyperthyroidism

Excessive production of thyroid hormone

Causes: Iodine overdose, thyroid hormone overdose, Graves' disease (key), tumors affecting the reproductive system

Symptoms: Skin color changes, weight loss, anxiety, possible goiter, nausea, exophthalmos, diarrhea, hair loss, elevated BP, fatigue, sweating

Tests: Elevated Systolic pressure noted, T3/T4 (free) levels increased, TSH levels reduced

Treatment: Radioactive iodine, surgery, beta-blockers, antithyroid drugs

Pharmacology Review

Drug Nomenclature

Generic name – Acetominophen

Trade name – TYLENOL, PANADOL

Routes of Drug Entry

Enteral

Oral: Easiest, safe, have 1st pass effect, large surface area for absoption, some medications irritate the GI, some medications may be degraded by the stomach.

Sub-lingual: Absorption through the oral mucosa with no 1st pass effect.

Rectal: Normally no 1st pass effect, usually used if patients are vomiting

Parenteral

Inhalation: Absorbed in the lungs, quick action, may cause inflammation in the lungs.

Injection (types):

- Intra-muscular: Easy access; may treat muscle or prolonged release into circulation.

- Subcutaneous: Injection just below the skin; causes a localized response. TB skin test.

- Intra-arterial: Used most commonly in chemotherapy also diagnostic procedures, drug introduced directly into the artery

- Intravenous: Can use an IV line, useful in emergencies, side effects appear quickly

- Intrathecal: Used with narcotic analgesics and local anesthetics. Drugs can reach the CNS and by-pass the blood brain barrier.

Drug Suffix	Example	Action
-azepam	Diazepam	Benzodiazepine
-azine	Chlorpromazine	Phenothiazine
-azole	Ketoconazole	Anti-fungal
-barbital	Secobarbital	Barbiturate
-cillin	Methicillin	Penicillin
-cycline	Tetracycline	Antibiotic
-ipramine	Amitriptyline	Tricyclic Anti-depressant
-navir	Saquinavir	Protease Inhibitor
-olol	Timolol	Beta Antagonist
-oxin	Digoxin	Cardiac glycoside
-phylline	Theophylline	Methylxanthine
-pril	Enalapril	ACE Inhibitor
-terol	Albuterol	Beta 2 Agonist
-tidine	Ranitidine	H_2 Antagonist
-trophin	Somatotrophin	Pituitary Hormone
-zosin	Doxazosin	Alpha 1 Antagonist

Cardiovascular pharmacology

Antiarrhythmics: Na+ channel blockers (Class I)

- *Class IA*: Procainamide, Disopyramide, Amiodarone, Quinidine
- *Class IB:* Mexiletine, Lidocaine, Tocainide
- *Class IC:* Flecainide, Encainide, Propafenone

Antiarrhythmics: (Beta blockers) (Class II) – Metroprolol, Atenolol, Propranolol Timolol, Esmolol

Antiarrhythmics: (K+Channel blockers) (ClassIII) – Sotaolol, Amiodarone, Bretylium, Ibutilide

Antiarrhythmics: (Ca2+ channel blockers) (Class IV) – Diltiazem, Verapamil

Vasodilators: Verapamil, Minoxidil, Hydralazine

Calcium Channel Blockers: Verapamil, Diltiazem, Nifedipine

Sympathoplegics: Beta blockers, Clonidine, Reserpine, Guanethidine, Prazosin

ACE Inhibitors: Lisinopril, Enalapril, Captopril

Cardiac glycosides: Digoxin

Dieuretics: Loop Dieuretics, Hydrocholorothiazide

K+ Sparing Dieuretics: Spironolactone, Triamterene, Amiloride

CNS Pharmacology

Sympathomimetics: Dopamine, Dobutamine, Epinephrine, Norephinephrine, Isoproterenol

Cholinomimetics: Carbachol, Neostigmine, Pyridostigmine, Echothiophate, Bethanechol

Cholinoreceptor blockers: Hexamethonium (nicotinic blocker), Atropine (muscarinic blocker)

Beta blockers: Atenolol, Nadolol, Propranolol, Metoprolol, Pindolol, Labetalol

Tricyclic Antidepressants: Doxepine, Imipramine, Amitriptyline, Nortriptyline, Amitriptyline

Parkinson's Treatment: L-dopa, Amantadine, Bromocriptine

Benzodiazepindes: Iorazepam, Triazolam, Oxazepam, Diazepam

Opiod Analgesics: Heroin, Methadone, Morphine, Codeine, Dextromethorphan, Meperidine

MAO Inhibitors: Tranylcypromine, Phenelzine

Seroton specific Re-uptake inhibitors: Paroxetine, Sertraline, Fluoxetine, Citalopram

Epilepsy Treatment: Valproic acid, Phenobarbital, Benzodiazepines, Gabapentin, Ethosuximide, Carbamazepine

Barbiturates: Pentobarbital, Thiopental, Phenobarbital, Secobarbital

IV Anethestics: Midazolam, Ketamine, Morphine, Fentanyl, Propofol, Thiopental

Local Anesthetics: Tetracaine, Procaine, Lidocaine

Neuroleptics (Antipsychotic drugs): Chlorpromazine, Thioridazine, Clozapine, Fluphenazine, Haloperidol

Alpha 1 Selective blockers: Terazosin, Prazosin, Doxazosin,

Alpha 2 Selective blockers: Yohimbine

Glaucoma Treatment: Prostaglandins, Dieuretics, Alpha agonists, Beta Blockers, Cholinomimetics

Cancer Treatment Drugs: Etoposide, Nitrosoureas, Cisplatin, Doxorubicin, Incristine Paclitaxel, Methotrexate, 6 – mercaptopurine, Busulfan, 5 – fluorouracil, Lomustine, Carmustine

Throbolytics: Urokinase, Anistreplase, Streptokinase, Alteplase

Cox 2 Inhibitors: Rofecoxib, Celecoxib

NSAID's: Naproxen, Indomethacin, Ibuprofen

Diabetic Treatment

Sulfonylureas: Chlorpropamide, tolbutamide, glyburide, Insulin (key), metformin

Glitazones: Rosiglitazone, Troglitazone, Pioglitazon

Asthma Treatment

Corticosteroids: Prednisone, Beclomethasone

Antileukotrienes: Zafirlukast, Zileuton

Beta 2 agonists: Salmeterol, Albuterol

Nonselective Beta agonists: Isoproterenolol

Muscarinic agonists: Ipratropium

H_2 blockers: Famotidine, Nizatidine, Cimetidine, Ranitidine

In-Depth Pharmacology Review

(Some of the drugs listed below fall outside an EMT's scope of practice. However, we have included them to help you in case a patient references these drugs.) If you have limited study time, focus on the cardiac, respiratory, and diabetic medications.

Cholinomimetrics

<u>Muscarinic Agonists</u>

Bethanecol (URECHOLINE): Increase GI motility

Carbachol (ISOPTO, MIOSTAT, CARBACHOL): Various types of glaucoma

Methacholine (PROVOCHOLINE): Test hyperactivity of airways

Pilocarpine: Used for glaucoma

<u>Anticholinesterases</u>

Anticholinesterases are used for Myasthenia gravis, glaucoma, and to increase tone in bladder.

- Physostigmine (ANTILIRIUM): Treat glaucoma, crosses BBB, reverse anticholinergic toxicity.
- Neostigmine (PROSTIGMIN): Synthetic form of Pysostigmine

Symptoms of Anticholinesterase toxicity: Miosis, rhinitis, cradycardia, GI spasms, bronchoconstriction, involuntary voiding of urine

Anticholinergics

<u>Muscarinic Antagonists and Ganglionic Blockers</u>

Muscarinic antagonists are used treat spastic GI, Parkinson's Disease, asthma, and treatment of peptic ulcers.

- *Atropine:* Anticholinergic (Parasympatholytics) effects; used in the treatment of renal colic, allergic rhinitis and peptic ulcers.
- *Scopolamine:* Causes cycloplegic, impotence and used primarily in motion sickness preparations

Ganglionic blockers

Examethonium: Blocks nicotinic receptors

Adrenegic agonists

Adrenegic Agonists (Sympathomimetics) are used to increase heart rate, and cause constriction of blood vessels. Used for shock treatment and cardiac decompensation.

Alpha-1 Selective agonists – Phenylephrine (NEO-SYNEPHRINE): Used to treat hypotension, tachycardia and nasal congestion.

Alpha-2 Selective agonists – Clonidine (CATAPRESS): Used as an antianxiety and analgesic drug. Also used to treat mild to moderate hypertension

Beta-1 Selective agonists

- Dobutamine (DOBUTREX): Short term management of cardiac decompensation following surgery
- Dopamine (DOPASTAT): Similar to Dobutamine

Beta-2 Selective agonists – Salbutamol (ALBUTEROL): Relaxes bronchial smooth muscle oral inhalant

Non-Selective Beta agonists Isoproterenol: Increases heart rate, vasodilation, bronchodilation, increased renin release

Mixed Alpha and Beta Agonists

> NE – (alpha 1 = alpha 2 > beta 1): Increased TPR, constriction of GI sphincters, elevates blood sugar

- ➢ Epinephrine: Increased systolic BP, decreased diastolic BP, bronchodilation, and relaxation of GI smooth muscles, also elevates blood sugar
- ➢ Amphetamines – Methylphenidate (RITALIN): Used to treat hyperactive disorders
- ➢ Ephedrine (EFEDRON NASAL): Used to treat shock, nasal congestion, asthma, narcolepsy

Adrenergic antagonists

Adrenergic Antagonists (Sympatholytics) are used in the treatment of migraines and vascular headaches.

Alpha-1 Antagonists used to decrease vascular tone and treatment of pheochromocytoma

- • Phenoxybenzamine (DIBENZALINE) used to treat Raynaud's disease
- • Prazosin (MINIPRESS) used to treat hypertension
- • Terazosin (HYTRIN) used to vasodilate and reduce serum lipid levels.

Non Selective Alpha antagonists

- • Phentolamine (REGITINE) control BP during pheochromocytoma
- • Ergot Alkaloids (Ergotamine) used to treat migraines and relax constricted vessels.

Beta-1 Blockers

- • Metoprolol (LOPRESSOR) used in the treatment of hypertension and blocks cardiac beta receptors
- • Atenolol (TENORMIN) used in the treatment of hypertension, chronic stable angina, and myocardial infarct

Non-Selective Beta Blockers (B1 and B2): Propranolol (INDERAL) prototype beta blocker used for the treatment of hypertension, angina, migraines, and to prevent MI

Centrally acting agents

Baclofen (LIORESAL): A derivative of GABA, used with spasticity. Side effects of transient drowsiness, confusion and hallucinations usually oral administration.

Benzodiasapines – Diazepam (VALIUM): Used with muscle spasms, some CP, cord lesions, side effects include sedation and physical addiction.

Direct acting relaxants

Dantrolene (DANTRIUM): Only drug with direct action on muscle cell used for severe spasticity. Side effects include hepatotoxic, and generalized muscle weakness.

Neuromuscular junction blockers (nmj)

Neuromuscular Junction Blockers are used with orthopedic procedures, tetanus poisioning, tracheal intubation and adjuvant in surgical anesthesia.

Depolarizing agents: Succinylcholine (ANECTINE) can paralyze muscle.

Non-Depolarizing agents: Curare or tubocurare

Side effects of (NMJ): Histamine release, malignant hyperthermia, breaks bones, elevated temperature. NMJ drugs are used to allow mechanical ventilation and intubation. Other examples include: Mivacurium chloride (Mivacron) and Pancuronium bromide (Pavulon).

Other muscle relaxants

Botulinum toxin (BOTOX) and Transdermal Clonidine

Local anesthetics

Benzocaine (AMERICAINE): Not absorbed through the skin, no systemic affect.

Lidocaine (XYLOCAINE): May cause drowsiness or tinnitis

Cocaine

Bupivicaine (MARCAINE): Epidural

Procaine (NOVOCAINE): Not used much

General anesthetics

Barbiturates (Thiopental – PENTOTHAL): Rapid onset, short acting.

Benzodiazapines (Diazepam – VALIUM)

Opiates (Meperidine – DEMEROL)

Sedative hypnotics

Barbiturates (Phenobarbital – SOLFOTON, NEMBUTAL, SECONOL): Reversibly depress activity in excitable membranes, hypnotic, and rapid tolerance. May cause residual CNS depression and contraindicated in the presence of pain.

Benzodiazapines: Used as a sedative, hypnotic, anti-anxiety, and anticonvulsant

Antianxiety agents

Benzodiazapines

Azapirones (BUSPAR)

Betablockers: Propranolol *(INDERAL)*

Alprazolam (XANAX)

Midazolam hydrochloride (VERSED)

Affective disorders

<u>Depression</u>

Tricyclics

- Amitriptyline (ELAVIL)
- Desipramine (PETOFRANE)
- Imipramine (JANIMINE)
- Doxepin (SINEQUAN)
- Clomipramine hydrochloride (Anafranil)

MAO Inhibitors – Phenelzine (NARDIL), Fluoxetine (PROZAC)

Second Generation Drugs (Side effects: sedation and insomnia)

- Fluoxetine (PROZAC)
- Sertraline (ZOLOFT)

<u>Manic Depression</u>

Lithium: Side effects include slurred speech, increased muscle tone, hand tremor, coma, confusion, nausea.

Antipsychotics

Phenothazines

- Chlorpromazine (THORAZINE)
- Thioridazine (MELLARIL)

Thioxanthines (high potency)

Butyrophenones – Haloperidol (HALODOL): Most common antipsychotic

Dihydroindolones

Dibenzoxazipines

- Loxapine (LOXITANE)
- Chlozapine (CLOZARIL)

Seizures

Partial: Simple, Carbamazepine, Phenytoin, Phenobarbital, Valproate

Complex: Carbamazepine, Phenytoin, Phenobarbital, Valproate

Partial progressing to General: Carbamazepine, Phenytoin, Phenobarbital, Valproate

Generalized:

- Absence (petit mal): Clonazepam, Ethosuximide, Valproate
- Myoclonic: Valproate
- Tonic/ Clonic: Carbamazepine, Phenytoin, Phenobarbital, Valproate
- Atonic: Clonazepam
- Status Epilepticus: Diazepam, Phenytoin, Phenobarb, Halothane

Opioids

Strong Agonists: Morphine, Meperidine (DEMEROL), Methadone (DOLOPHINE).

Mild to moderate Agonists: Codeine (CODEINE SULFATE)

Mixed Agonists and Antagonists: Butorphanol (STADOL)

Antagonists: Naloxone (NARCAN)

Side Effects of Opioids: Euphoria, sedation, OH, respiratory depression

Non-opioid analgesics

General: (NSAIDs) non steroidal anti-inflammatory drugs

Salicylates – Aspirin: Used to treat fever, prevent DVT, prevent coronary artery thrombus, treat mild to moderate pain including headache, and muscle aches Side effects include GI damage, hepatotoxicity, renal toxicity, salicylate overdose, Reye's Syndrome, Aspirin allergy. Other NSAIDs are Ibuprofen (ADVIL, MOTRIN), Indomethacin (INDAMETH, INDOCIN).

Acetominophen (Tylenol): Not an NSAID

Anti-inflammatory drugs

Steroids – Cortisol: Commonly used with spinal cord injury, organ transplants, asthma, COPD, and rheumatic disorders (RA, Lupus). Side effects include immunosupression, cataract formation, alters fluid and electrolyte balance, myopathy.

- Prednisolone (PRELONE)
- Prenisone (DELTASONE)
- Dexamethasone (DEXASONE)

Histamine Antagonists: Decrease bronchospams, decrease edema and itching. Decrease capillary permeability, decrease vasoconstriction.

- 1st Generation Drugs
  - "amine" suffix: Diphenhydramine (BENADRYL), Chlorpheniramine (CHLOR-TRIMETON), Pyrilamine (NISAVAL), Carbinoxamine (CARDEC)
  - "izine" suffix: Hydroxyzine (ATARAX), Cyclizine (MAREZINE), Promethazine (PHENERGAN)
- 2nd Generation Drugs (Do not cross blood brain barrier): "adine" suffix, Loratadine (CLARITIN), Terfenadine (SELDANE)

Respiratory pharmacology

Antitussives: Suppress cough may contain NSAIDS. Side effects includesedation, GI distress and dizziness

- Benzonatate (TESSALON)
- Dextromethorphan (various trade names)
- Hydrocodone (HYCODAN), TRIAMINIC)
- Codeine (various trade names)

Decongestants: Most commonly alpha agonists. Side effects include headache, dizziness, nervousness and nausea.

- Ephedrine (PRIMATENE tabs)
- Epinephrine (PRIMATENE MIST)
- Oxymetazoline (AFRIN)
- Phenylephrine (NEO SYNEPHRINE)
- Pseudoephedrine (ACTIFED, SUDAFED)

Antihistamines: Adjunct in asthma, not real effective if used alone, decreased nasal congestion. Used for the treatment of rhinitis, motion sickness and idiopathic urticaria. Side effects include sedation, dizziness, blurred vision, and incoordination.

- Chlorpheniramine (CHLOR-TRIMETON)
- Clemastine (TAVIST)
- Loratidine (CLARATIN)
- Terfenadine (SELDANE)
- Doxylamine (UNISOM NIGHT TIME SLEEP AID)
- Dimenhydrinate (DRAMAMINE)
- Diphenhydramine hydrochloride (BENADRYL)
- Cetirizine hydrochloride (ZYRTEC)

Mucolytics: ecrease mucous viscosity used to treat the common cold to pneumonia. Side effects include GI distress and inflammation of oral mucosa.

- Acetylcysteine (MUCOMYST, MUCOSIL) primary drug

Expectorants: Increase respiratory secretions, increase ejection of mucous. Side effects include GI distress.

- Guaifenesin (ROBITUSSIN): Primary medication

Obstructive Pulmonary Disease

- Beta-agonists: Side effects include bronchia irritation with prolonged use.
- Xanthines (Theophlline, Theobromine): Side effects include nausea, confusion, seizures, irritability
- Anti-cholinergics: Side effects include dry mouth, tachycardia, blurred vision, confusion
- Anti-inflammatory
  - Corticosteroids: Side effects include osteporosis, muscle wasting, cataracts and hypertension
  - Cromolyn Sodium: Blocks histamine from mast cells. Side effects include nasal and respiratory irritation.
  - Leukotriene Antagonists – Montelukast (SINGULAR): Side effects include fatique, fever, GI, dizziness and headache

Gi pharmacology

Antacids (TUMS, ROLAIDS, MILK of MAGNESIA): Attempt to neutralize acids. Used in the treatment of hyperacidity, indigestion, hyperphosphatemia, esophageal reflux, peptic ulcers and gastric ulcers.

H2 Blockers (TAGAMENT, PEPCID, AXID, ZANTAC): Block histamine reactions on GI, used for ulcers

Antidiarrheal medications
- Opioids (PAREGORIC): Decrease GI motility
- Absorbents (KAOPECTATE): Sequester the toxic product causing the diarrhea. Holds the harmful bacteria and toxins.
- Bismuth salicylate (PEPTO-BISMOL): Decreases GI secretions, stimulate water absorption in the large intestine.

Emetics (Apomorphine, Ipecac): Induces vomiting by stimulating the medullary emetic center.

Antiemetics: Antihistamines, phenothiazines (anti-psychotics), anticholinergics (Scopalamine). Antiemetics are used to decrease inner ear sensitivity and stimulate vomiting.

Cholelitholytics: Used to dissolve gallstones

Electrolytes – (Mg2+), (Ca2+), (HCO$_3$), (K+), (Na+): Used in the treatment of hyponatremia, hypokalemia, hypocalcemia and metabolic acidosis.

Acid/Base Modifiers

- Alkalinizers: Increase alkalinity and used in the treatment of metabolic acidosis. Examples include Sodium lactate, Sodium bicarbonate, and Tromethamine

- Acidifiers: Increase acid levels and used in the treatment of metabolic alkalosis. Example: ammonium chloride

Laxatives: Used for constipation. Laxatives may include stimulants, fecal softeners, or saline substances.

Cardiovascular pharmacology

BP = CO x SVR

Classes of Antihypertensives: Presynaptic agents (centrally acting, peripherally acting), Dieuretics, Beta Blockers, Alpha Blockers, Vasodilators, Calcium Entry Blockers, Angiotensin Converting Enzyme (ACE) Inhibitors

Diuretics: Side effects include metabolic disorders, reflex tachycardia, vasoconstriction, orthostatic hypotension, decreased cardiac contractility. Antidieuretics are used in the treatment of postoperative distention and diabetes insipidus. Diuretics are used in the treatment of kidney disease, heart failure and endocrine disorders. Types of diuretics:

- Thiazide diuretics: Chlorthiazide (DIURIL), Hydrochlorothiazide (ESIDRIX), Benzthiazide (HYDREX, EXNA)

- Loop Diuretics: Bumetadine (BUMEX), Ethacrynic Acid (EDECRIN), Furosemide (LASIX, FUROSIDE)
- K sparing Diuretics block K secretion at distal tubule: Amiloride (MIDAMOR), Spironolactone (ALDACTONE), Triamterene (DYRENIUM)

Beta blockers: Decrease HR and force contraction
- Non selective – Propranolol (INDERAL)
- B1 selective – Atenolol (TENORMAN)
- Mixed antagonist/agonist Labetalol (NORMODYNE)

Alpha Blockers: Used only in severe hypertension, now used more frequently in mild to moderate hypertension. Side effects includereflex tachycardia and orthostatic hypotension
- Doxazosin (CARDURA)
- Phenoxybenzamine (DIBENZYLINE)
- Proazosin (MINIPRESS)
- Terazosin (HYTRIN)

Presynaptic Inhibitors: Side effects include orthostatic hypotensin and GI distress.
- Reserpine (SERPALAN)
- Guanethidine (ISMELIN

Centrally Acting Agents – alpha 2 agonists, decrease Sympathetic Nervous System outflow from CNS. Side effects include dizziness, drowsiness, and dry mouth.
- Clonidine (CATAPRES)
- Guanabenz (WYTENSIN)
- Methyldopa (ALDOMET)

Vasodilators: Side effects include reflex tachycardia, dizziness, postural hypotension, weakness, GI distress, fluid retention, hirsutism.

- Hydralazine (APRESOLINE)
- Minoxidil (LONITEN)
- Diazoxide (HYPERSTAST)
- Nitroprusside (NITROPRESS)

ACE inhibitors: Side effects include allergy, GI distress, dizziness, chest pain and non productive cough.

- Captopril (CAPOTEN)
- Benazepril (LOTENSIN)

Calcium Channel Blockers: Block entry of Ca into Vascular Smooth Muscle and/or cardiac muscle. Side effects include excessive vasodilation, nausea, dizziness, abnormal HR, orthostatic hypotension.

- Nifedipine (PROCARDIA)
- Verapamil (CALAN, ISOPTIN)
- Diltiazem (CARDIZEM)

Angina Pectoris

- Organic Nitrates: Vasodilators – Decrease cardiac preload, and afterload. Side effects include headache, dizziness, orthostatic hypotension, and nausea. Examples are Nitroglycerin (NITRO-BID, NITROSTAT) and Amyl Nitrate
- Beta Blockers: Decrease H.R., force of contraction. Side effects include cardiac depression and asthmatics beward. Examples are Atenolol (TENORMIN), and Propranolol (INDERAL).
- Calcium Entry Blockers (CEBs): Vasodilate coronaries, general vasodilation. Side effects include headache, edema, dizziness, disturbance of cardiac rhythm, orthostatic hypotension, and fatigue. Examples are Diltiazam (CARDIZEM), Nifedipine (PROCARDIA).

Cardiac Arrhythmias: Ued in the treatment of paroxysmal atrial tachycardia, ventricular tachycardia, PVC's, and atrial fibrillation.

- Class I Drugs: Side effects include aggravation of rhythm disturbances, dizziness, nausea, visual disturbances
  - ➤ Class 1A – Quinidine (CARDIOQUIN), Procainamide (PROMINE)
  - ➤ Class 1B – Lidocaine (XYLOCAINE): Severe ventricular arrhythmias
  - ➤ Class 1C – Ecainide (ENKAID)
- Class II Drugs- Beta Blockers: Decrease cardiac contractility and prolong refractory period, best for supraventricular arrhythmias (AV node), and some ventricular arrhythmias
- Class III Drugs – Bretylium (BRETYLOL): Used for ventricular arrhythmias. Side effects include transient increase in arrhythmias, orthostatic hypotension.
- Class IV Drugs – Calcium Entry Blockers: Side effects include excessive bradycardia and peripheral vasodilation. Verapamil is the most effective; Diltiazam is somewhat effective.

CHF: Excessive fluid accumulation, blood backs up into capillaries

Left Heart Failure	Right Heart Failure
L Heart doesn't pump adequately	R Ht. Doesn't pump adeq.
Fluid backs up in lungs	Peripheral back up (blood)
Pulmonary Edema	Peripheral Edema
Shortness of Breath	

Cardiac Glycosides: Increase intracellular calcium, stabilizes heart rate and slows impulse conduction. Side effects include GI distress, drowsiness, fatigue, confusion, ventricular fib.

Diuretics: Decrease fluid volume and therefore edema. Side effects include fatigue, confusion, and nausea.

ACE Inhibitors

Others: Amrinone and Milrinone – Increase myocardial contractility

Dopamine/Dobutamine: Sometimes used in acute heart failure- not used often, only in advanced cases or non-responsives

Vasodilators: Used for severe heart failure- will cause hypotension, may include alpha blockers and direct vasodilators

Inotropics: Used in the treatment of atrial flutter, CHF, Paroxysmal atrial tachycardia, and atrial fibrillation.

Coagulation/blood disorders

Anticoagulants: Prevent excessive clot formation in the VENOUS system. Used in the treatment of pulmonary embolism, cerebral accident, and malabsorption syndrome.

- Heparin: Must give parenterally (IV or SubQ), set indwelling need (heparin lock) for IV
- Warfarin: Impairs livers ability to synthesize clotting factors; given orally and has a lag time of 2 days

Antithrombotics: Dipyridamole (Dipridacot) and Sulfinpyrazone (Antuvane) – Used in the prevention of MI, and to prevent thromboembolism following arterial surgery like coronary bypass and arterial grafts.

Thrombolytics: Streptokinase and Urokinase, Tissue Plasminogen Activator, and Antistreplace (Eminase): Used to Breakdown existing clots, used with pulmonary embolism and to open clogged bypass shunts, also used with acute MI if given within 3-6 hours. Side effects include hemorrhage, back or joint pain, GI distress, hypersensitivity, and fever.

Hematics: Used in the treatment of pernicious anemia and megaloblastic anemia to increase the number of RBC's.

Hyperlipidemia

HMG-CoA Reducatase Inhibitors: Lovastatin (Mevacor) and Prevastatin (Prevachol) – Inhibit the enzyme used in early step of cholesterol synthesis.

Fibric Acids: Clofibrate (Abitrate) and Genfibrozil (Lopid) – Breakdown of LD

Others

- Cholestyramine: (QUESTRAN) – Increases excretion of bile acids, cholesterol
- Niacin: (VIT B3) – Inhibits production of VLDL
- Probucol: (LORELCO) – Breaks down LDL and inhibits deposition into arterial wall

Diabetes mellitus

Insulin: All type I, some type II, have rapid, short acting preps (for uncontrolled diabetes), have intermediate and long acting preps for better controlled. All injections, cannot take orally- all protein digested in GI

Oral hypoglycemics: (Sulfonylureas) – Give orally to decrease blood glucose in type II not type I, increases release insulin, increases sensitivity of cells to insulin. Adverse effects include hypoglycemia, heartburn, GI distress, and headache

Glucagon: Given to treat hypoglycemia; adverse effects include nausea, vomiting, and allergic reaction.

Cyclosporine: (Sandimmune) – Immunosuppresant may help protect against beta cell destruction if given soon after onset of symptoms (type 1); long term success not known.

- Aldose Reductase Inhibitors
- Biquanides: Decrease production of gluocose, used with Type II Diabetes
- Meglitinide Insulin: Used with Type II Diabetes, (glucose dependent)

Key signs of Hypoglycemia: Confusion, fatigue, inappropriate sweating, nausea, hunger, anxiety, and tachycardia

Controlled Substance Categories

Schedule I	Highest potential abuse, used mostly for research. (heroin, peyote, marijuana)
Schedule II	High potential abuse, but used for therapeutic purposes (opioids, amphetamines and barbiturates)
Schedule III	Mild to moderate physical dependence or strong psychological dependence on both. (opioids such as codeine, hydrocodone that are combined with other non-opoid drugs)
Schedule IV	Limited potential for abuse and physical and/or psychological dependence (benzodiazepines, and some low potency opioids)
Schedule V	Lowest abuse potential of controlled substances. Used in cough medications and anti-diarrheal preps.

Dose Response: The relationship between dose and the body's response is called a dose-response curve (DRC).

Potency: Relates to the dosage required to produce a certain response. A more potent drug requires a lower dosage than does a less potent drug to produce a given effect.

Efficacy: Usually refers to maximum efficacy. Maximum efficacy is plateau (or maximum response), but may not be achievable clinically due to undesirable side effects. In general, the steepness of the curve dictates the range of doses that are useful therapeutically.

LD_{50}/ED_{50}: Quantal dose response curve is the relationship between the dose of the drug and the occurrence of a certain response.

Therapeutic index (TI): The ratio of the median effective dose (ED_{50}) and the toxic dose (TD_{50}) is a predictor of the safety of a drug. This ratio is called the therapeutic index. Note: Acetominophin has TI of 27. Meperidine (DEMEROL) has a TI of 8.

Psychological Terms

Empathy: Capacity to understand what your patient is experiencing from that patient's perspective.

Defense mechanisms

Compensation: Covering up a weakness by stressing a desirable or strong trait

Denial stage: The second reaction stage of psychologic adjustment to physical disablement or loss; an unconscious defense mechanism in which existence of unpleasant realities is blocked from conscious awareness

Displacement: Transferring of an emotion, or actual loss of function as a result of illness or accident

Projection: Attributing of our own unwanted trait onto another person

Rationalization: The justification of behaviors using reason other than the real reason

Reaction Formation: A defensive reaction, in which a behavior is exactly the opposite of what is expected

PTSD (Posttraumatic stress disorder): Psychopathologic reaction to a traumatic event

Lability: Emotional instability; manifested by alterations or fluctuations in emotional state.

Dysphoria: Exaggerated feelings of depression; may be accompanied by anxiety

Perseveration: A patient continues to repeat a movement, word or expression, even though it is meaningless. Associated with TBI or brain damage

Anxiety: Feelings of apprehension associated with the following sympathetic reactions; increased heart rate, dyspnea, hyperventilation, dry mouth and GI symptoms (nausea/vomiting).

Grief process

Denial: Patients insist they are fine, joke about themselves or are not motivated to participate in the treatment

Anger: Patients may become disruptive, blame others and do not admit to any improvement. The defense mechanism of displacement may occur.

Bargaining: Patients may turn to religion or others in charge and make promises to affect a return of function or any further loss of function

Depression: Patients may withdraw, cry or lose interest in treatment. Motivation is low and needs to be monitored closely by the P.A.. The patient has an overwhelming sense of loss.

Acceptance: Patients have worked through other grief stages, accepted their condition, relate more to their treatment and make plans for the future.

Conditions

Alzheimer's Disease: Chronic, progress, widespread deterioration of the cerebrum. There is intellectual decline, loss of memory, confusion, anxiety, depression, loss or reasoning, possible motor impairment, and gait problems as the disease progresses.

Bipolar disorder (manic-depressive): Disorder characterized by mood swings from depression to mania. In the manic phase, patients often present with intense outbursts, high energy and activity, excessive euphoria, decreased need for sleep, and unrealistic beliefs.

Conversion Disorder: Response to severe emotion stress resulting in involuntary disturbance of physical functions

Depressive reaction: Neurotic reaction to a personal loss or failure that is disproportionate in intensity and duration

Pathological Conditions

AIDS: Caused by a retrovirus in which viral RNA becomes part of the host cell DNA. Reduction in T-cells (<250) and a high viral load can cause HIV to progress to AIDS. Low immunity can lead to opportunistic infections like pneumoncystsis carinnii, secondary cancers, salmonella, neuropathies, and meningitis. Use of protease inhibitors in combination with other drugs seems to be a major step in the management of HIV.

Cellulitis: Inflammation of the connective tissue, tends to be widespread and is poorly defined. It is frequently accompanied by infection. The skin over the area is often hot, red, and edematous, and resembles the skin of an orange.

CHF: May result in tachycardia, decreased stroke volume, LE swelling and decreased cardiac output.

Cystic fibrosis: Thickening of secretions of all exocrine glands, leading to obstruction. Probable multiple frequent respiratory infections especially Staph. Aureus and Pseudomonas Aeruginosa

Dermatitis: Superficial inflammation of the skin, characterized by vesicles (when acute), redness, edema, oozing, crusting, scaling and usually itching

Deep vein thrombosis: Formation of an abnormal blood clot in a deep vein. If the clot breaks free it may become a pulmonary embolus. Symptoms include a +Homan's sign, positive doppler. Anticoagulant therapy is indicated in most cases.

Diabetes Mellitus Insulin dependent: Due to the absolute insulin deficiency and can lead to diabetic ketoacidosis.

Diabetes mellitus-non-insulin-dependent diabetes: Usually associated with obesity and is caused by a combination of insulin resistance and a defect in beta-cell responsiveness to elevated plasma glucose concentration. Plasma insulin concentration is usually normal or elevated.

Down's syndrome Trisomy 21: Altered facial appearance, intellectual disability, simian crease, congenital heart disease

Duchenne's muscular dystrophy: X-linked recessive disease with noted pelvic weakness and calf hypertrophy.

Gout: Metabolic disease marked by elevated level of serum uric acid and deposition of urate crystals in the joints, soft tissue and kidneys. Treatment often involves anti-inflammatory medications, daily use of colchicine and lowering of urate concentration in body fluids with diet.

Hemophilia: Bleeding disorder that is inherited and has to do with clotting factor deficiency.

Hepatitis: Inflammation of the liver and may be caused by viral or bacterial infections or chemical agents. Transmission is from blood, body fluids, or body tissues, through oral or sexual contact or contaminated needles. Signs/Symptoms include elevated lab values of hepatic transaminases and bilirubin, enlarged liver with tenderness, fever and jaundice. Treatment-IV fluids, analgesics, interferon and vaccines

Herpes zoster: Acute nervous system viral infection involving the dorsal root ganglia and characterized by vesicular eruption and neuralgic pain I the cutaneous areas supplied by peripheral sensory nerves arising at the infected dermatome or myotome. Treatment involves corticosteroids for pain relief in many cases.

Intermittent claudication: Arterial insufficiency that results in ischemia to the exercising muscle. Relief of pain is achieved by resting.

Psoriasis: Chronic disease of the skin with erythematous plaques covered with a silvery scale; common on the scalp, elbows, knees, and genitalia. Treatment involves long-wave UV light, combination UV light with oral photosensitizing drug (Psoralen).

Pulmonary embolism: Athrombus from the peripheral venous circulation lodges in the pulmonary artery with the subsequent obstruction of blood flow to the lungs. Treatment often involves a low-dose heparin, analgesis, and pulmonary vasodilators.

Rhematoid arthritis: Complaints of fatigue, weight loss, weakness and general diffuse musculoskeletal pain are often the initial presentations. Pain is localized to specific joints with symmetrical bilateral presentation. Deformities of the fingers are common.

Reye's syndrome (hepatoencephalophathy): Sometimes fatal with children related to viruses and aspirin.

Systemic lupus erythematosus: Chronic, systemic rheumatic, inflammatory disorder of the connective tissues which affects multiple organs including skin and joints.

Tuberculosis: Infection spread by droplets from the untreated infected host. Treatment involves medications to eliminate infection.

Wilson's Disease (hepatolenticular degeneration): Copper does not enter circulation and builds up in the brain, liver and eye.

Major hormones

Growth hormone: Major stimulus of postnatal growth: Induces precursor cells to differentiate and secrete insulin-like growth factor I which stimulates cell division, stimulates protein synthesis

Insulin: Stimulates fetal growth, stimulates postnatal growth by stimulating secretion of IGF-1, stimulates protein synthesis

Thyroid hormones: Permissive for growth hormone's secretion and actions, permissive for development of the central nervous system

Testosterone: Stimulates growth at puberty, in large part by stimulating the secretion of growth hormone, causes eventual epiphyseal closure, stimulates protein synthesis

Estrogen: Stimulates the secretion of growth hormone at puberty, causes eventual epiphyseal closure

Cortisol: Inhibits growth, stimulates protein catabolism

Digestive System

Digestion is a process that food is absorbed. The mouth begins to prepare food for digestion. Teeth grind food into smaller substrates. Then salivary glands, which secrete saliva, begin digestion of the food using enzymes. The pharynx and esophagus allow passage of the food into the stomach. The stomach uses gastric juices and absorbs a small amount of the food. Then, the food goes to the small intestine. The pancreas and the liver release enzymes and bile respectively into the small intestine to aid in absorption. The small intestine is composed of the duodenum, jejunum, and ileum. Then, substrates are passed into the large intestine, which has little digestive function. Absorption of water and electrolytes does occur in the large intestine.

Peristalsis is the wave like movement occurring in the digestive system that propels food downward. The alimentary canal is the path food travels from the mouth to the anus. Feces are composed mostly of water and substrates and are not absorbed.

Key terms

Cholelithiasis: Stones in the gallbladder

Diverticulitis: Inflammation of the small pouches in the colon, if present

Hepatitis: Inflammation of the liver

Stomatitis: Inflammation of the mouth

Dyspepsia: Indigestion

Enteritis: Inflammation of the intestine

Ear

The external ear collects sound and passes the sound to the tympanic membrane. Then the middle ear increases the force of the sound waves using the malleus, stapes, and incus. Auditory tubes connect the middle ear to throat and help maintain proper pressure. The inner ear consists of complex system of tubes and chambers-osseous, membranous labyrinths and also the cochlea. Auditory impulses are interpreted in the temporal lobes.

Eye

The wall of the eye has an outer, middle and inner layer. The sclera (outer layer) is protective. The cornea refracts light entering the eye and is found on the anterior aspect of the sclera. The choroid coat (middle layer) helps keep the inside of the eye dark. The retina (inner layer) contains the receptor cells. The visual receptors are rods and cones. Rods are responsible for colorless vision in dim light, and cones are responsible for color vision.

Key terms

Otitis media: Inflammation of the middle ear

Diplopia: Double vision

Tinnitus: Ringing in the ears

Vertigo: Sensation of dizziness

Reproductive System

Male reproductive organs are specialized for the formation of sperm (gamete) and transporting sperm. The vas deferens is the tube that sperm travels through. Semen is composed of sperm cells and secretions of the prostate and bulbourethral glands. Semen activates sperm cells.

Testosterone is the most important male hormone. Testosterone encourages the development of male sex organs. It is responsible for the development of male secondary sexual characteristics.

Female reproductive organs are specialized for childbirth and development of a fetus. The primary structures are the ovaries, uterus, and vagina. The ovaries release an egg cell (gamete) into the uterus. The uterus sustains life for the embryo until childbirth. The vagina allows transportation of the fetus during delivery.

Estrogen and progesterone are the primary female sex hormones. Estrogen is responsible for female sexual characteristics. Progesterone is responsible for changes in the uterus. Menopause is related to low estrogen levels and changes in the female reproductive organs. The product of fertilization is a zygote with 46 chromosomes.

Key terms

Amenorrhea: Absence of menstrual flow

Gestation: 40 weeks of pregnancy

Orchitis: Inflammation of a testis

Cesarean section: Birth of a fetus through an abdominal incision

Urinary System

The urinary system consists of the kidneys, ureters, bladder, and urethra. The kidney functions to remove metabolic wastes from the blood and excrete them. The also help regulate blood pressure, pH of the blood, and red blood cell production. The basic functional unit of the kidney is the nephron. The nephron consists of a renal corpuscle and a renal tubule. Urine is the end product of the urinary system. The kidneys are involved in filtration, re-absorption and secretion. Glomerular filtration is regulated by osmotic pressure.

The ureter is a tube that connects the kidneys and the bladder. Kidney stones can become lodged in the ureter. Peristaltic waves in the ureter force urine to the bladder. The bladder stores urine and forces urine into the urethra. Muscle fibers in the wall of the bladder form the detrusor muscle.

Key terms

Enuresis: Uncontrolled urination

Dieuretic: A substance that encourages urination

Pyuria: Pus in the urine

Ureteritis: Inflammation of the ureter

Amniocentesis: Removal of some fluid surrounding the fetus for analysis. Fetus location is identified by US prior to the procedure. Results may take a month.

Chorionic villus sampling: Removal of placental tissue for analysis from the uterus during early pregnancy. US helps guide the procedure. 1-2 weeks get the results. Can be performed earlier than amniocentesis.

Preeclampsia: Presence of protein in the urine, and increased BP during pregnancy. Found in 8% of pregnancies.

Eclampsia: Seizures occurring during pregnancy, symptoms of pre-eclampsia have worsened. Factors that cause eclampsia vs. pre-eclampsia relatively unknown.

Oligohydramnios: Low levels of amniotic fluid that can cause: fetal abnormalities, ruptured membranes and fetus disorders.

Polyhydamnios: High levels of amniotic fluid that can cause: gestational diabetes and congenital defects.

Breast infections/Mastitis: Infection or inflammation due to bacterial infections. (S. aureus).

Cervicitis: Infection, foreign bodies, or chemicals that causes inflammation of the cervix.

Pelvic inflammatory disease: Infection of the fallopian tubes, uterus or ovaries caused by STD's in the majority of cases.

Toxic shock syndrome: Infection of (S. aureus) that causes organ disorders and shock.

Maternal Responses to Pregnancy

Breasts: Enlarge and develop mature grandular structure. cause: Estrogen, progesterone, prolactin, and placental lactogen

Blood Volume: Increases cause: total erythrocyte volume is increased by erythropoietin and plasma volume by salt and water retention

Calcium balance-positive: The cause is increased parathyroid hormone and 1,25 dihydroxyvitamin D3

Body weight: Increases by an average of 12.5 kg, 60 percent of which is water

Circulation-Cardiac output increases, total peripheral resistance decreases (vasodilation in uterus, skin, breasts, GI tract, and kidneys), mean arterial pressure stays constant

Respiration: Hyperventilation (arterial PCO2 decreases)

Organic metabolism: Metabolic rate increases.

Appetite and thirst: Increase

Nutritional RDA's: Increase

Initial Assessment of Burns

Initial assessment

1. ABC's
   - *Airway:* If inhalation injury is suspected, a bonchoscopy may be indicated to determine extent of injury. Endotracheal tube placement early in order to avoid tracheostomy and complications. Tracheostomy bypasses upper respiratory system. Primary responsibility for the EMT-I is maintaining the airway.
   - *Breathing:* Caution if burn wound is circumferential partial to full thickness in the region of the chest. Escharotomy may be indicated to facilitate excursion of the chest wall. Escharotomy is a longitudinal incision through eschar and down to subcutaneous tissue. An Escharotomy would be performed at a trauma center or ER.
   - *Circulation:* Control bleeding from internal trauma, fractures, etc. Caution if burn wound is circumferential, partial to full thickness involving an extremity as vascular occlusion may result. Escharotomy may be indicated in order to restore blood perfusion. Persistent edema involving an extremity may lead to compartment syndrome. Clinical presentation includes numbness, poor capillary refill, decreased pulse and temperature and pallor. Fasciotomy would be indicated.
2. Complete evaluation process to determine extent and depth of burn.
3. Shock: The most immediate life-threatening complication due to moderate-severe burn wound injury. Hypovolemia is a loss of circulatory fluids into interstitial spaces. Clinical presentation is decrease in BP, decreased urinary output,

and an increase in hematocrit. Intravascular fluid is the first fluid to be depleted, followed by interstitial fluid while the most stable is intercellular fluid. Treatment includes hydration with IV fluids via two large-bore 16 gauge needles. Amount of fluid administered is based upon TBSA/body weight via Parkland/Baxter formula. Excessive hydration may result in cerebral, pulmonary edema.

Wound care terms

Maceration: Process of becoming soft or separated into constituent elements or as if by steeping in fluid.

Eschar: Scab formed after a burn; may be thick, leathery or thin appearing white to beize or green.

Necrosis: Localized death of living tissue. Devitalized, avascular, dehydrated and may appear brown to black.

Slough: A mass of dead tissue separating from an ulceration; appears loose, stringy; usually white to beige often associated with infection.

Induration: To increase the fibrous element; to make hard as in the presence of cellulitis.

Rubor: Red; erythema

Calor: Heat

Dolor: Pain

Tumor: Hard or indurated

Erythema: Abnormal redness of the skin due to capillary congestion

Pitting edema: An abnormal excess accumulation of serous fluid in connective tissue. Palpation of the area creates an indentation in the soft tissue.

Hypergranulation: Excessive amount of granulation tissue which retards epithelialization; red beefy in color

Hypogranulation: Excessive amount of epithelial tissue which grows down into the wound cavity and retards granulation; pink and shiny. Also known as proud flesh.

Dehiscence: To split the lines or borders of an incision

Transudate: Water and electrolytes (clear)

Exudate: Protein and leukocytes (cloudy)

Serous: Clear fluid found within blisters. Formed following coagulation and contains immune bodies

Sanguineous: Consisting of or relating to blood

Serosanguineous: Combination of clear and bloody drainage

Lavage: Therapeutic washing of an organ

Excoriation: To wear off the skin, abrade, denude.

Denude: To strip off all covering

Purulent: Containing or consisting of pus; white blood cells.

Desiccated: To dry up; dehydrate

Undermining: A separation or space between the periwound skin and the sidewall of the wound bed.

Skeletal System

Axial skeleton

The axial skeleton consists of 80 bones forming the trunk (spine and thorax) and skull.

Vertebral Column

The main trunk of the body is supported by the spine, or vertebral column, which is composed of 26 bones, some of which are formed by the fusion of a few bones. The vertebral column from superior to inferior consists of 7 cervical (neck), 12 thoracic and 5 lumbar vertebrae, as well as a sacrum, formed by fusion of 5 sacral vertebrae, and a coccyx, formed by fusion of 4 coccygeal vertebrae.

Ribs and Sternum

The axial skeleton also contains 12 pairs of *ribs* attached posteriorly to the thoracic vertebrae and anteriorly either directly or via cartilage to the *sternum* (breastbone). The ribs and sternum form the *thoracic cage*, which protects the heart and lungs. Seven pairs of ribs articulate with the sternum (*fixed ribs*) directly, and three do so via cartilage; the two most inferior pairs do not attach anteriorly and are referred to as *floating ribs*.

Skull

The skull consists of 22 bones fused together to form a rigid structure which houses and protects organs such as the brain, auditory apparatus and eyes. The bones of the skull form the *face* and *cranium* (brain case) and consist of 6 single bones (*occipital, frontal, ethmoid, sphenoid, vomer* and *mandible*) and 8 paired bones (*parietal, temporal, maxillary, palatine, zygomatic, lacrimal, inferior concha* and *nasal*). The *lower jaw* or *mandible* is the only movable bone of the skull (head); it articulates with the temporal bones.

Other Parts

Other bones considered part of the axial skeleton are the *middle ear bones* (*ossicles*) and the small U-shaped *hyoid bone* that is suspended in a portion of the neck by muscles and ligaments.

Appendicular skeleton

The *appendicular skeleton* forms the major internal support of the appendages—the *upper* and *lower extremities* (limbs).

Pectoral Girdle and Upper Extremities

The arms are attached to and suspended from the axial skeleton via the *shoulder* (*pectoral*) *girdle*. The latter is composed of two *clavicles* (*collarbones)* and two *scapulae* (*shoulder blades*). The clavicles articulate with the sternum; the two *sternoclavicular joints* are the only sites of articulation between the trunk and upper extremity.

Each upper limb from distal to proximal (closest to the body) consists of hand, wrist, forearm and arm (upper arm). The *hand* consists of 5 *digits* (fingers) and 5 *metacarpal* bones. Each digit is composed of three bones called *phalanges*, except the thumb which has only two bones.

Pelvic Girdle and Lower Extremities

The lower *extremities*, or legs, are attached to the axial skeleton via the *pelvic* or *hip girdle*. Each of the two coxal, or *hip bones* comprising the pelvic girdle is formed by the fusion of three bones—*illium, pubis,* and *ischium*. The coxal bones attach the lower limbs to the trunk by articulating with the sacrum.

THE HUMAN SKELETAL SYSTEM	
Part of the Skeleton	**Number of Bones**
Axial Skeleton	**80**
Skull	22
Ossicles (malleus, incus and stapes)	6
Vertebral column	26
Ribs	24
Sternum	1
Hyoid	1
Appendicular Skeleton	**126**
Upper extremities	64
Lower extremities	62

Characteristics of Bone

Bone is a specialized type of connective tissue consisting of cells (*osteocytes*) embedded in a calcified matrix which gives bone its characteristic hard and rigid nature. Bones are encased by a *periosteum*, a connective tissue sheath. All bone has a central marrow cavity. *Bone marrow* fills the marrow cavity or smaller marrow spaces, depending on the type of bone.

Compact and spongy bones

There are two types of bone in the skeleton: *compact bone* and *spongy* (cancellous) bone.

- *Compact bone* lies within the periosteum, forms the outer region of bones, and appears dense due to its compact organization. The living osteocytes and calcified matrix are arranged in layers, or *lamellae*. Lamellae may be circularly arranged surrounding a central canal, the *Haversian canal*, which contains small blood vessels.

- *Spongy bone* consists of *bars, spicules* or *trabeculae*, which forms a lattice meshwork. Spongy bone is found at the ends of long bones and the inner layer of flat, irregular and short bones. The trabeculae consist of osteocytes embedded in calcified matrix, which in definitive bone has a lamellar nature. The spaces between the trabeculae contain bone marrow.

Bone Cells

The cells of bone are osteocytes, osteoblasts, and osteoclasts.

- *Osteocytes* are found singly in *lacunae* (spaces) within the calcified matrix and communicate with each other via small canals in the bone known as *canaliculi*. The latter contain osteocyte cell processes. The osteocytes in compact and spongy bone are similar in structure and function.

- *Osteoblasts* are cells which form bone matrix, surrounding themselves with it, and thus are transformed into osteocytes. They arise from undifferentiated cells, such as mesenchymal cells. They are cuboidal cells which line the trabeculae of immature or developing spongy bone.

- *Osteoclasts* are cells found during bone development and remodeling. They are multinucleated cells lying in cavities, *Howship's lacunae*, on the surface of the bone tissue being resorbed. Osteoclasts remove the existing calcified matrix releasing the inorganic or organic components.

Bone Matrix

Matrix of compact and spongy bone consists of collagenous fibers and ground substance which constitute the organic component of bone. Matrix also consists of inorganic material which is about 65% of the dry weight of bone. Approximately 85% of the inorganic component consists of calcium phosphate in a crystalline form (hydroxyapatite crystals). Glycoproteins are the main components of the ground substance.

Major types of bones

Type of Bone	Characteristics	Examples
Long bones	Width less than length	Humerus, radius, ulna, femur, tibia
Short bones	Length and width close to equal in size	Carpal and tarsal bones
Flat bones	Thin flat shape	Scapulae, ribs, sternum, bones of cranium (occipital, frontal, parietal)
Irregular bones	Multifaceted shape	Vertebrae, sphenoid, ethmoid
Sesamoid	Small bones located in tendons of muscles	---------

Joints

The bones of the skeoeton articulate with each other at *joints*, which are variable in structure and function. Some joints are immovable, such as the *sutures* between the bones of the cranium. Others are *slightly movable joints*; examples are the *intervertebral joints* and the *pubic symphysis* (joint between the two pubic bones of the coxal bones).

Joint Type	Characteristic	Example
Ball and socket	Permits all types of movement (abduction, adduction, flexion, extension, circumduction); it is considered a universal joint.	Hips and shoulder joints

Hinge (ginglymus)	Permits motion in one plane only	Elbow and knee, interphalangeal joints
Rotating or pivot	Rotation is only motion permitted	Radius and ulna, atlas and axis (first and second cervical vertebrae)
Plane or gliding	Permits sliding motion	Between tarsal bones and carpal bones
Condylar (condyloid)	Permits motion in two planes which are at right angles to each other (rotation is not possible)	Metacarop-phalangeal joints, temporomandibular

Adjacent bones at a joint are connected by fibrous connective tissue bands known as *ligaments*. They are strong bands which support the joint and may also act to limit the degree of motion occurring at a joint.

EMT-P Exam Facts

1. C3-C5 spinal levels corresponds for the phrenic nerve which activates the diaphragm.

2. Safety should be your primary responsibility at the scene of an accident for yourself and co-workers.

3. Increased ICP can lead to Cushing's Triad; which involves increased BP, decreased pulse and Cheyne-Strokes respirations.

4. If you are correcting a documentation error, put your initials and the date next to the single strike through line for error correction.

5. Appendicitis can cause tenderness at McBurney's points just superior to the right iliac crest.

6. Take vital signs every 5 minutes with critical patients. Every 15 minutes with non-critical patients.

7. Good Samaritan laws will protect you if you are acting within your scope of practice.

8. If you have cleared the patient's cervical spine the head tilt-chin lift is the best way to get the airway open.

9. Large pupils are considered dilated and small pupils are considered constricted.

10. Delivery of oxygen via nasal cannula at 40% = 6LPM

11. Taking a history of a patient should involve the acronym SAMPLE: S-Signs/Symptoms, A-Allergies, M-Medications, P-Past medical history, L-Last oral food/drug, E-Event causing call.

12. If a reporter asks you the name of an accident victim, do not give them the victim's name. You must observe patient confidentiality.

13. IO insertion is contraindicated with fractures of the legs.

14. Know the METTAG system – Triage.

15. A drop in Systolic pressure by at least 10 mmHg is called pulsus paradoxus.

16. Kidney stones can cause sharp lateral pain and vomiting.

17. Establish scene safety before beginning the ABCs.

18. EMT-B's provide BLS, EMT-I's provide ALS

19. Bunker gear is required involving traumatic accidents. (Gloves, Eye Wear protection, Helment and Proper Clothing).

20. The correct dose of aspirin for individuals having a heart attack is 162-325 mg.

21. Pediatric patients suffering from an allergic reaction are often given Benadryl – 1 mg/kg.

22. Pediatric patient suffering from cardiac arrest should be given Epinephrine .01 mg/kg

23. Pediatric patient suffering from ventricular tachycardiac can be given 5 mg/kg of amiodarone.

24. Pediatric patient suffering from opiate toxicity should be given .1mg/kg Naloxone.

25. Damage to the anterior aspect of the eye involving blood perfusion can be considered- Hyphema

26. Cushing syndrome is treated with sodium bicarbonate in many cases.

27. If a child is having a medical emergency, the parent cannot refuse EMT services for the child.

28. The dive reflex causes blood to centralize in the body and BP to drop.

29. LSD and Heroin are Schedule I drugs.

30. Elevated ICP can lead to Biot's respiratory pattern

31. TB is transferred via airborne droplets.

32. A minor cannot refuse care by himself or herself.

33. The tipe of a blade used to intubate an adult client should be in contact with the epiglottis.

34. Decerebrate posturing-arms and legs extended.

35. Decorticate posturing-(flexion noted)

36. Pursed-lipped breathing is indicated for people with COPD

37. APVU- Alert, Responds to verbal, Response to pain, Unresponsive

38. Know the Glasgow Coma Scale- 15= normal score, <8 Head Injury Severe

39. If an individual is showing signs of Hypotension do not give Nitroglycerin.

40. Atropine is given in cases were an individuals cardiac signs and symptoms are extremely unstable.

41. PVC's that are bigeminal are often treated with 1 mg/kg of Lidocaine

42. If you are following the pulseless electrical activity algorithm you should give Epinephrine first.

43. You can be accused of battery if you touch someone inappropriately.

44. Heat cramps are the first indicator of heat exhaustion.

45. Acute pulmonary edema is often treated with Lasix to decrease fluid volumes.

46. The maximum time limits for suctioning are 15 sec-adult and 5 sec-peds case.

47. ECG strip time for a small block is .04 sec. For a large block .20 seconds.

48. CISM- Critical incident stress management

49. OSHA- Occupational Safety and Health Administration

50. FCC- Federal Communications Commission

51. START- Simple Triage and Rapid Response

52. START Key Points: 1. Walk 2. Respirations 3. Pulse 4. Neurological condition

53. If cardiac ischemia is present dopamine is contraindicated due to vasopressor qualities.

54. The right atrium contains the SA node

55. Ventricular fib is treated with: Lidocaine, Vasopressin, and Epinephrine

56. Never give Lidocaine to patients with severe AV or SA blocks.

57. Visceral pleura covers the lungs.

58. The thoracic cavity is covered by parietal pleura.

59. Beck's triad-Neck veins bulging, Hypotension, poor heart sounds

60. Murphy's sign- gallbladder pain near the right costal inferior margin.

61. QRS complex normal time is .08 sec to .12 sec

62. Never use a tourniquet below the knee or elbow.

63. Abdominal aortic aneurysm – may show a palpable mass that is pulsating.

64. Individuals with asthama that has progressed to a severe condition can be treated with subcutaneous epinephrine.

65. Grey-Turner's sign- lateral ecchymosis presentation

66. Check the carotid artery in the neck in adults if they are unconscious. Check the radial artery if they are conscious.

67. Normal range of Phenergan is 12.5 to 25 mg per dose.

68. Prior to mechanical capture millivolts are increased steadily with transcutaneous pacing.

Practice Test

Practice Questions

1. Which of the following statements regarding allergies is **FALSE**?

   a. A type I allergic reaction can be life-threatening

   b. Immunity can be natural or acquired

   c. Anaphylactoid reactions are mediated by an antigen-antibody reaction

   d. Immunity can be artificially induced

2. All of the following patients are at high risk of latex allergy **except**

   a. Tollbooth operators

   b. Asthmatics

   c. Hairdressers

   d. Patients with allergic rhinitis

3. You are called by the husband of a 25-year-old woman who has developed a severe allergic reaction to shellfish. On arrival, the woman's face is swollen, and hives appear on her arms and legs. She complains of tightness in her neck and has difficulty breathing. The first step in treating this patient is to

   a. Administer IV epinephrine

   b. Transport the patient to the hospital

   c. Administer high-concentration oxygen

   d. Administer IV saline solution

4. All of the following drugs may be given safely in addition to epinephrine **except**

   a. Beta agonists

   b. Beta-blockers

   c. Antihistamines

   d. Corticosteroids

5. Which of the following is **NOT** a typical sign of an allergic reaction?

   a. Urticaria

   b. Diarrhea

   c. Bronchoconstriction

   d. Altered mental status

6. In performing defibrillation, the paddles should be placed

   a. Over the sternum

   b. Over the pacemaker

   c. To the right of the upper sternum and to the left of the left nipple

   d. To the left of the upper sternum and to the right of the right nipple

7. In performing defibrillation, the following may be used to decrease paddle-skin interface resistance

   a. Creams used in ECG monitoring

   b. Pads soaked in alcohol

   c. Pads soaked in water

   d. Pads soaked in saline

8. In performing defibrillation, you should

   a. Remove nitroglycerin patches before defibrillation

   b. Place the paddles together before firing the defibrillator

   c. Alternate cardiopulmonary resuscitation with defibrillation

   d. Perform open air discharge of the defibrillator to remove an unwanted charge

9. Which of the following statements regarding asynchronous cardiac pacing is **FALSE**

    a. Asynchronous pacing is typically used in asystole

    b. Asynchronous pacing may be used to control dysrhythmia

    c. Asynchronous pacemakers are used more frequently than demand pacemakers

    d. The asynchronous mode may be used to determine heartbeat in cases of electrocardiogram interference

10. Transcutaneous cardiac pacing should be used in

    a. Patients with open wounds

    b. Bradycardia

    c. Cardiac arrest

    d. Pulseless electrical activity

11. According to American Hospital Association guidelines, in which of the following cases is resuscitation appropriate?

    a. Presence of a DNAR order

    b. Septic shock

    c. Asystole

    d. Drug overdose

12. Which of the following statements regarding biphasic defibrillation is **FALSE**?

    a. Biphasic defibrillation of 115 J is equivalent to 200 J monophasic defibrillation

    b. Initial defibrillation should be 4 J/kg for a pediatric patient

    c. Initial defibrillation should be at 360 J monophasic energy

    d. The optimal current for ventricular defibrillation is 30 to 40 A

13. You are called to the home of an 88-year-old woman suffering from an acute pulmonary episode. The patient complains of extreme dyspnea. She is sitting upright but leaning forward and breathing through pursed lips; wheezing and rhonchi are evident. Initial assessment of this patient indicates that she is suffering from

   a. COPD

   b. Asthma

   c. ARDS

   d. Pneumonia

14. The signs and symptoms in the patient described above are indicative of

   a. Pneumonia

   b. Bronchitis

   c. Emphysema

   d. Asthma

15. Typical signs and symptoms of chronic bronchitis include

a. Nonproductive cough

b. Pink or red complexion

c. Chronic cyanosis

d. Pursed-lip breathing

16. All of the following are indicated in treatment of a patient in respiratory distress **except**

   a. Establishing an IV line

   b. Applying a cardiac monitor

   c. Pulse oximetry

   d. Withholding oxygen

17. Which of the following letters in the acronym OPQRST used in obtaining a history of a patient in respiratory distress is **INCORRECT**?

    a. O = onset

    b. S = sensitivity

    c. P = provocation

    d. Q = quality

18. Which of the following is indicative of a perfusion problem?

    a. Asthma

    b. Atherosclerosis

    c. Shock

    d. Carbon monoxide poisoning

19. Which of the following statements regarding obstructive airway disease is **TRUE**?

    a. A patient can manifest COPD and asthma at the same time

    b. Patients with emphysema are referred to as "blue bloaters"

    c. Patients with chronic bronchitis are referred to as "pink puffers"

    d. Childhood asthma usually persists throughout adulthood

20. The wife of a 50-year-old man calls for assistance for her husband, who is having a severe asthma attack. On arrival, the patient is in respiratory distress, with loud and rapid respirations and audible wheezing. The patient's wife states that he has recently discontinued corticosteroid therapy. After administering oxygen, the next step should be to

    a. Administer CPAP

    b. Administer albuterol

    c. Administer BiPAP

    d. Administer ketamine

21. Inspiratory wheezing in the patient described above may indicate

 a. Upper airway occlusion

 b. Respiratory failure

 c. Secretions in the large airways

 d. Pneumonia

22. A PEFR test is most often used

 a. In patients in severe respiratory distress

 b. In children less than 5 years of age

 c. Before drug administration

 d. In patients with ARDS

23. The sister of an 85-year-old woman calls for assistance, stating that she thinks her sister is having a stroke. On arrival, the patient is conscious but slightly confused and her speech is slurred. Her sister states that a few moments ago, the patient appeared disoriented and did not seem to recognize her own name; she also has a history of hypertension. The patient states that she feels better and does not want to go to the hospital. Proper initial treatment for this patient should include

 a. Managing hypertension

 b. Establishing time of symptom onset and transporting

 c. Administering anticoagulant therapy

 d. Performing a CT scan

24. All of the following are useful in the diagnosis of stroke **except**

 a. CPSS

 b. LAPSS

 c. Medical history

 d. 50% Dextrose

25. The following statements regarding TIAs are true **except**

  a. The signs and symptoms of a TIA are the same as those of stroke

  b. A TIA is the most important predictor of a brain infarction

  c. TIAs are associated with permanent neurological damage

  d. Initial assessment of a patient with a TIA is the same as that of a stroke victim

26. You are called to the home of a 40-year-old woman complaining of severe "gas pains" and cramps in her stomach. On arrival, the patient is lying on the couch, holding her lower abdomen. She states that she was experiencing severe cramping in her lower abdomen, with profuse sweating and nausea; the pain progressed in severity but has now subsided. The first step in caring for this patient is to

  a. Conduct an initial scene survey

  b. Offer pain medication

  c. Transport to the hospital

  d. Perform a complete physical examination

27. In using the mnemonic OPQRST to obtain a history of abdominal pain, the letter P stands for

  a. Pain onset

  b. Pain severity

  c. Past medical history

  d. Provocation

28. Which of the following would NOT be considered in obtaining a SAMPLE history for the patient described above?

  a. Change in bowel habits

  b. Regularity of menstrual periods

  c. Pain location

  d. Last meal or oral intake

29. An example of a condition associated with visceral pain is

    a. Cholecystitis

    b. Peritonitis

    c. Ulcer

    d. Morphine addiction

30. After obtaining a thorough patient history from the patient described in Question 26, you find that she has had 2 or 3 previous episodes of cramping pain, increasing in intensity, then quickly subsiding. Pain radiates to the right upper quadrant and usually occurs at night, especially after consuming fried or fatty foods. This patient is probably suffering from

    a. Pancreatitis

    b. Cholecystitis

    c. Crohn's disease

    d. Bowel obstruction

31. Which of the following statements regarding nasogastric intubation is **FALSE**?

    a. Nasogastric intubation is indicated in cases of abdominal distention

    b. Nasogastric intubation may be associated with gastrointestinal bleeding

    c. Nasogastric intubation is not indicated in unconscious patients

    d. Nasogastric intubation is indicated only under medical direction

32. All of the following statements regarding dialysis are true **except**

    a. Dialysis patients with chronic renal failure cannot tolerate increased potassium levels

    b. Dialysis may be associated with dysrhythmias

    c. Dialysis patients are at increased risk of hemorrhage

    d. Peritoneal dialysis is slower than hemodialysis

33. In treating graft occlusion associated with thrombosis in a patient with acute or chronic renal failure, you should

    a. Irrigate the graft

    b. Clear the graft by aspiration

    c. Obtain the blood pressure in the extremity with an arteriovenous graft

    d. Administer fluids intravenously in an alternative site

34. In the case of poisoning, gastric lavage is indicated

    a. Before tracheal intubation

    b. After tracheal intubation

    c. In adults only

    d. 2 to 3 hours after ingestion

35. Which of the following statements regarding gastric lavage is **FALSE**?

    a. Gastric lavage is contraindicated in the case of gasoline ingestion

    b. Gastric lavage is contraindicated in the case of ingestion of caustic agents

    c. Only water should be used for gastric lavage in pediatric patients

    d. Only normal saline should be used for gastric lavage in pediatric patients

36. All of the following statements regarding use of syrup of ipecac are true **except**

    a. Syrup of ipecac is suitable for routine use in the out-of-hospital setting only

    b. Syrup of ipecac is contraindicated in patients with altered consciousness

    c. Syrup of ipecac is contraindicated in pregnancy

    d. Syrup of ipecac is commonly found in patients' homes

37. The antidote for calcium channel blockers is

    a. Bicarbonate

    b. Ethanol

    c. Calcium

    d. Glucagon

38. The mother of a 2-year-old boy calls to report her son has ingested most of a small bottle of baby oil. On arrival, the child is crying, with a loud hacking cough. His mother states that he spontaneously vomited after swallowing the contents of the bottle. The first line of treatment for this child is to

    a. Decontaminate the stomach

    b. Administer activated charcoal

    c. Administer syrup of ipecac

    d. Provide a patent airway

39. An example of a hydrocarbon associated with significant toxicity is

    a. Asphalt

    b. Baby oil

    c. Tar

    d. Grease

40. Which of the following symptoms is associated with methanol poisoning?

    a. Cyanosis

    b. Hemolytic anemia

    c. Bacterial pneumonia

    d. Blindness

41. Which of the following plants is **NOT** poisonous?

    a. Mistletoe

    b. Buttercups

    c. Marigold

    d. Daffodil

42. Which of the following is **NOT** indicated in treatment of cyanide poisoning associated with smoke inhalation?

    a. Cyanide antidote kit

    b. Amyl nitrate

    c. Hydroxocobalamin

    d. Oxygen

43. The principal treatment for tick bite is

    a. Nail polish

    b. Isopropanol

    c. Burning match

    d. Tick removal

44. Benzodiazepines are used to treat overdose of

    a. Tricyclic antidepressants

    b. Heroin

    c. Cocaine

    d. PCP

45. Diazepam is **NOT** indicated in overdose of

    a. Antipsychotics

    b. Opioids

    c. Cocaine

    d. Lysergic acid diethylamide or LSD

46. Which of the following statements regarding treatment of drug-induced cardiovascular emergencies is **FALSE**?

    a. Naloxone is used in treating meperidine-induced seizures

    b. Benzodiazepines are used in treating acute coronary syndrome

    c. Benzodiazepines are used in treating acute anticholinergic syndrome

    d. Naloxone is used in treating opioid poisoning

47. Treatment of drug-induced ventricular fibrillation may include

    a. High-dose epinephrine

    b. Propranolol

    c. Electrical defibrillation

    d. Calcium

48. Which of the following is NOT a major mechanism of heat loss?

    a. Convection

    b. Absorption

    c. Radiation

    d. Conduction

49. The manager of a golf course calls to report that a 65-year-old man has collapsed after playing golf for several hours in 100º F heat. The patient did not seem to be aware of his surroundings and began talking to himself shortly before collapsing. On arrival, the patient is conscious but suffering from convulsions; his skin is flushed and his core body temperature (CBT) is increased. After initiation of BLS and ALS measures, proper treatment for this patient should be to

    a. Submerge the patient in ice water

    b. Administer large quantities of fluids

    c. Remove the patient's clothing

    d. Cover the patient with blankets and transport

50. A common symptom of heat stroke is

    a. Profuse sweating

    b. Absence of sweating

    c. Electrocardiogram changes

    d. Increased muscle tone

51. All of the following are indicated in the treatment of hypothermia **except**

    a. Passive rewarming

    b. Removing the patient's clothing

    c. Active internal rewarming

    d. Active external rewarming

52. Which of the following is a clinically significant factor in the care of a drowning victim?

    a. Aspiration of contaminants

    b. Dry drowning

    c. Wet drowning

    d. Duration of submersion

53. Which of the following is **NOT** significant in pressure-related diving emergencies?

    a. Henry's law

    b. Newton's law

    c. Dalton's law

    d. Boyle's law

54. Acute mountain sickness may result in

  a. Coma

  b. Cough with frothy sputum

  c. Altered consciousness

  d. Impaired memory

55. According to Centers for Disease Control (CDC) guidelines, in the absence of blood, universal precautions for prevention of HIV transmission do **NOT** apply to exposure to

  a. Semen

  b. Amniotic fluid

  c. Vomitus

  d. Synovial fluid

56. Which of the following statements regarding HCV infection is **FALSE**?

  a. HCV is often transmitted through sexual contact

  b. HCV infection most often results from needle-stick injury

  c. No vaccine has been developed for HCV

  d. Most patients with HCV are asymptomatic

57. You are called to a homeless shelter to assist a 42-year-old man whose severe coughing is "disrupting" the other residents. On arrival, an emaciated man is coughing violently and wiping his mouth with a handkerchief. He complains of fatigue and states that he has been coughing up blood. He admits to being HIV-positive, but states that he has never had any type of lung disease. This patient is most likely suffering from

  a. HCV

  b. TB

  c. Pneumonia

  d. HBV

58. Which of the following statements regarding TB infection is **FALSE**?

   a. TB is more prevalent in patients with HIV infection

   b. Residents of homeless shelters are at high risk of TB

   c. TB can be transmitted by coughing or sneezing

   d. The most common form of TB transmission is through the skin or mucous membranes

59. To prevent the transmission of TB to the paramedic, all of the following are required by the National Institute for Occupational Safety and Health (NIOSH) **except**

   a. Surgical mask

   b. N-type respirator

   c. HEPA filter

   d. Respiratory protection program

Questions 60 and 61 refer to the following scenario:

   The mother of a 4-year-old boy calls you, stating that her son has been projectile vomiting and has a "bad rash" on his foot. On arrival, the boy says he has a "bad headache" and a "stiff neck." He has a low-grade fever, and a petechial rash is visible.

60. The most likely diagnosis in this patient is

   a. Rubella

   b. Measles

   c. Tetanus

   d. Meningitis

61. Treatment of the patient should include all of the following **except**

    a. BSI precautions

    b. Placement of a surgical mask

    c. Antibiotics

    d. Analgesics

62. Which of the following statements regarding rabies infection is **FALSE**?

    a. An animal suspected of carrying rabies should be killed

    b. Rabies vaccine is given by a series of injections in the stomach

    c. Rabies infection may result in eye and facial muscle paralysis

    d. Tetanus prophylaxis may be indicated for rabies

63. Which of the following statements regarding SARS is **TRUE**?

    a. The majority of SARS cases improve spontaneously

    b. Quarantine is no longer required for SARS patients

    c. SARS is usually transmitted via close contact with family members or coworkers

    d. SARS may be transmitted via blood transfusion

64. Which of the following statements regarding bird flu is **FALSE**?

    a. Bird flu may be transmitted by pigs

    b. Bird flu may be transmitted among humans

    c. Bird flu may be transmitted among different bird species

    d. Antiviral therapy is not indicated for bird flu prophylaxis

65. Which of the following is **NOT** part of the recommended procedure for transport of SARS patients?

    a. Used needles should be collected in sharps containers

    b. Non-patient areas of the vehicle should also be cleaned

    c. Paramedics who may have been exposed to SARS after patient transport may continue working

    d. Compressed air may be used to clean the vehicle and any reusable equipment

Questions 66 and 67 refer to the following scenario:

    The brother of a 30-year-old man calls to request assistance because his brother is "completely out of control." On arrival, the patient is pacing around the room and shouting obscenities. His brother states that the patient had been throwing objects around the room and had threatened to "kill somebody." He also states that the patient had been treated in the past for "manic-depression" but discontinued taking his medication because he had been sick with the flu. You observe a bottle of vodka on the table.

66. In assessing this patient, you should first

    a. Conduct a brief physical examination

    b. Restrain the patient and transport to the hospital

    c. Interview the patient

    d. Contact the police for assistance

67. While interviewing the patient, he suddenly accuses you of "interrogating" him and begins throwing objects around the room. To manage this situation, you should first

   a. Offer the patient a last chance to cooperate

   b. Call the police and leave the scene

   c. Apply chemical restraint

   d. Restrain the patient using wrist restraints

68. All of the following agents are useful in chemical restraint **except**

   a. Haloperidol

   b. Diazepam

   c. Lithium

   d. Diphenhydramine

69. In caring for a victim of sexual assault, which should be done first?

   a. Examine the patient's genitalia

   b. Obtain a sexual history

   c. Move the patient to a separate room

   d. Remove and bag the patient's clothing for law enforcement

70. You are called to the scene of a severe traffic accident involving a 25-year-old pregnant woman. The woman is 6 months pregnant and has sustained significant head trauma. Your first priority in managing this patient is to

   a. Assess fetal heart rate

   b. Administer high-concentration oxygen

   c. Transport the patient in the supine position

   d. Apply a pneumatic antishock garment

71. Treatment of third-trimester bleeding should include all of the following **except**

    a. IV fluid therapy

    b. Measurement of fundal height

    c. Vaginal examination

    d. Administration of high-concentration oxygen

72. Which of the following should **NOT** be used to determine the need for resuscitation of a baby just born?

    a. Apgar score

    b. Muscle tone

    c. Crying

    d. Amniotic fluid

73. All of the following should be used to stimulate uterine contraction following delivery **except**

    a. Administering oxytocin

    b. Packing the vagina to control bleeding

    c. Massaging the uterus

    d. Encouraging breastfeeding

74. Which of the following is an example of safe ambulance operation?

    a. Using high beams to increase visibility

    b. Using a police escort in response to an emergency call

    c. Using lights and sirens to provide absolute right of way

    d. Using warning devices during transport of a patient with life-threatening injury

75. The 2-second rule should be applied in gauging braking distance for

    a. Larger emergency vehicles

    b. Poor roadway conditions

    c. Type III emergency vehicles

    d. Heavy vehicle weight

76. Which of the following statements regarding air medical services is **FALSE**?

    a. Ground ambulances are faster than air ambulances within a 30-mile range in urban areas

    b. Fewer crashes occur with air than with ground ambulances

    c. Fewer individuals survive helicopter crashes

    d. Air ambulances can accommodate more patients and equipment

77. You arrive at the scene of a crash of a small chartered plane. Two of the passengers are conscious and have sustained minor injuries; one has broken his arm in several places. A third passenger is unconscious, with a carotid pulse but not a radial pulse. The pilot has suffered significant head trauma with severe hemorrhage and has a respiratory rate of less than 10 breaths per minute. The primary line of treatment for these patients is to

    a. Administer epinephrine

    b. Set any broken limbs

    c. Reposition the airway and control hemorrhage

    d. Treat for hypovolemia

78. The START technique is used for

    a. Assessing the airway

    b. Primary triage

    c. Critical incident stress management

    d. Secondary triage

79. Proper treatment for the passenger with the broken arm described above would be to

    a. Direct the patient to remain at the scene for further assistance

    b. Assess the patient's respiratory rate

    c. Evaluate the patient's mental status

    d. Check the patient's pulse rate

80. In the case of the passenger described above with a carotid pulse but no radial pulse, you should

    a. Assess mental status

    b. Classify as delayed

    c. Classify as critical

    d. Classify as dying

81. During a blizzard, a commuter plane crashes into a river, submerging all of the passengers; the water temperature is 35ºF. All of the following rescue techniques are valid **except**

    a. Lifting victims onto a back board

    b. Directing multiple passengers to huddle together

    c. Directing a single passenger to assume the fetal position

    d. Putting on a PFD before rescue

82. Which of the following statements regarding hypothermia is **FALSE**?

    a. Rapid hypothermia can improve brain viability

    b. The effectiveness of the cold protective response depends on age

    c. Resuscitation should not be attempted after prolonged submersion in extremely cold water

    d. Sudden exposure to extremely cold water can lead to laryngospasm

83. In the case of a confined-space emergency,

    a. Use the SCBA as an air supply

    b. Obtain a copy of the OSHA permit

    c. Shoring is required for all cave-ins

    d. Approach the lip of the cave-in to assess the scene

84. During a severe thunderstorm, a car is hit by downed electrical wires, trapping the two passengers inside. Proper management of this situation should include

    a. Securing the downed wires

    b. Extricating the passengers from the vehicle

    c. Instructing the passengers to remain inside the vehicle

    d. Instructing the passengers to climb out the back window

85. In rescuing an accident victim in an airbag-equipped car, you should

    a. Disconnect the car battery if the airbag is deployed

    b. Maintain a safe distance of 20 inches for passenger-side airbags

    c. Turn on the ignition to test whether the battery is disconnected

    d. Place a hard board between the passenger and the airbag

86. During a high-angle rescue attempt, which of the following is mandatory?

    a. ALS

    b. Endotracheal intubation

    c. Supplemental oxygen

    d. IV line

87. Tactics for paramedic safety in the course of a potentially violent situation include all of the following **except**

    a. Avoidance

    b. Tactical retreat

    c. Confrontation

    d. Concealment

88. A bulletproof vest is **NOT** effective against

    a. Knives

    b. Ice picks

    c. Handgun bullets

    d. Airgun pellets

89. Which of the following is useful for protection against hazardous materials?

    a. SCBA

    b. Air-purifying respirator

    c. Level C clothing

    d. Level D clothing

90. You are called to the scene of a hazardous chemical spill caused by an overturned truck. On arrival, the truck driver has suffered severe leg trauma; the drivers and passengers of nearby vehicles were not seriously injured. Proper emergency treatment of the truck driver should include

    a. Wound debridement

    b. Removal from the hot zone

    c. IV therapy

    d. Spinal immobilization

91. Following a hazardous materials or "hazmat" incident, proper procedure should include all of the following **except**

a. Showering to remove potential contaminants

b. Leave the incident immediately and continue to the next emergency

c. Hazmat establishment of a decontamination corridor

d. Debriefing of rescue personnel

92. Which of the following statements regarding pediatric anatomy is **FALSE**?

a. Children have a larger body surface area-to-body mass ratio

b. A child in shock may maintain a normal blood pressure

c. The liver and spleen are less often injured in children

d. In children, the muscles provide the primary means of support for the chest wall

93. In assessing a 5-year-old girl who is not acutely ill, the paramedic should

a. Monitor vital signs every 5 minutes

b. Allow the child to play with the stethoscope

c. Conduct a physical exam from toe to head

d. Obtain an electrocardiogram reading

94. The mother of a 4-year-old boy calls at 2 AM to report that her son has awakened with "a terrible cough and trouble breathing." On arrival, the child is sitting upright in bed and coughing; nasal flaring and slight cyanosis are present. The mother states that the child has had a "bad cold" over the last 2 weeks and is running a low fever. This child is likely suffering from

a. Croup

b. Epiglottitis

c. Pneumonia

d. Airway obstruction

95. Proper management of the child described above should include

    a. Intubation

    b. Parenteral antibiotics

    c. Bronchodilators

    d. Cool humidified air

96. Treatment of status epilepticus in a child may include all of the following **except**

    a. Diazepam

    b. Glucagon

    c. Intubation

    d. Cardiac monitoring

97. Which of the following is **NOT** indicated in the emergency treatment of a child with hyperglycemia?

    a. IV fluid therapy

    b. Insulin

    c. Glucose testing

    d. Dextrose

98. A possible cause of SIDS is

    a. Suffocation

    b. Regurgitation

    c. Allergies

    d. Upper airway obstruction

99. You are called to the apartment of an 85-year-old woman complaining of shortness of breath, pain in her right calf, and a "racing heart." The patient states that she has a history of CHF. On examination, tachycardia and tachypnea are present, as well as mild edema of the right calf. This patient is most likely suffering from

a. Bacterial pneumonia

b. Pulmonary embolism

c. Myocardial infarction

d. Heart failure

100. Aggressive airway management, including supplementary oxygenation and IV bronchodilator therapy, is indicated in

a. COPD

b. Cerebral vascular disease

c. Pulmonary embolism

d. Bacterial pneumonia

101. Sudden disorientation, with incoherent speech, mental confusion, and excitement, is associated with

a. Alzheimer's disease

b. Dementia

c. Delirium

d. Senility

102. Which of the following statements regarding trauma management of elderly patients is **FALSE**?

a. PaO_2 decreases with age

b. Rapid fluid IV administration is indicated in elderly patients

c. Elderly patients may require higher arterial pressures for perfusion

d. Adjustment of stroke volume may be decreased in response to hypovolemia

103. The rule of nines is useful for

a. Infants

b. Irregularly shaped burns

c. Burns over a large area of the body

d. Children over 10 years of age

104. A moderate burn may be classified as

a. A full-thickness burn covering greater than 10% of body surface area

b. A partial-thickness burn covering 15% of body surface area

c. A burn from contact with a caustic chemical

d. A burn from contact with high-voltage electricity

105. In managing a burn victim, the paramedic should

a. Apply ointment to the burn

b. Remove blisters already formed

c. Cover the patient with a sterile blanket

d. Place an ice pack on the burn

106. The sister of a 20-year-old woman calls to report that she has found her sister in the family car with the windows rolled up and the heat on. The young woman is semi-conscious and has been in the car for about 3 hours. Her sister states that the young woman has been depressed because of the break-up of a serious relationship. Proper treatment of this patient may include all of the following **except**

    a. High-concentration oxygen

    b. Pulse oximeter

    c. Sodium thiosulfate

    d. Hyperbaric oxygen

107. In the patient described above, the most appropriate line of action following medical care is to

    a. Transport the patient immediately

    b. Question the patient's sister about the patient's medical history

    c. Ask the patient directly about suicidal intent

    d. Call law enforcement

108. A carbon monoxide blood level of 10% produces

    a. No symptoms

    b. Electrocardiogram abnormalities

    c. Coma

    d. Nausea and vomiting

109. Increasing intracranial pressure may be controlled by

    a. IV fluid therapy

    b. The Valsalva maneuver

    c. Blood replacement therapy

    d. Osmotic diuretics and steroids

110. All of the following may be used to determine left ventricular function **except**

   a. PCWP

   b. RAP

   c. LAP

   d. PAP

111. Which of the following drugs increases respiration?

   a. Diazepam

   b. Aspirin

   c. Epinephrine

   d. Morphine

112. The following drug may be safely given to a pregnant woman:

   a. Morphine

   b. Aspirin

   c. Diazepam

   d. Oxytocin

113. Drugs that are given during pregnancy only if the potential benefit justifies the risk to the fetus are classified as

   a. Category X

   b. Category B

   c. Category C

   d. Category D

114. The nasal cannula is typically used in patients with

   a. Apnea

   b. Chest pain

   c. Hypoxia

   d. Respiratory insufficiency

115. Which of the following devices may be used in patients with apnea?

   a. Bag-mask device

   b. Nasal cannula

   c. Partial nonbreather mask

   d. Nonbreather mask

116. Which of the following statements regarding rescue breathing is **FALSE**?

   a. The jaw-thrust technique is used in patients with suspected spinal injury

   b. Use of an oropharyngeal or nasopharyngeal airway is contraindicated in an unconscious patient

   c. Mouth-to-stoma ventilation is more sanitary than the mouth-to-mouth technique

   d. The mouth-to-nose technique requires the patient's mouth to be closed

117. The bag-mask device should **NOT** be used to

   a. Provide supplemental oxygen to a spontaneously breathing child

   b. Provide ventilation to a child in respiratory arrest

   c. Provide ventilation under extreme environmental temperatures

   d. Provide ventilation to a patient who has not been intubated

118. Nasal airways may be used in all of the following cases **except**

   a. Unconsciousness

   b. Cervical spine injuries

   c. Seizures

   d. Fractured skull

119. Cuffed endotracheal tubes may be indicated for

   a. Infants

   b. Children 8 to 10 years old or older

   c. Children less than 8 years old

   d. Adults only

120. Which of the following statements regarding blind intubation is **FALSE**?

   a. Blind intubation may be necessary in disaster situations involving many victims

   b. Blind intubation is indicated when the airway cannot be visualized

   c. Nasotracheal intubation is a blind procedure

   d. Blind intubation is indicated in patients with spinal fractures

121. An inaccurate pulse oximeter reading may result from

   a. Cyanosis

   b. Spinal injury

   c. Nail polish

   d. Hypertension

122. In-line stabilization is required for intubation of

   a. Infants

   b. Children under the age of 10

   c. Patients with hypertension

   d. Patients with spinal injuries

123. Use of the LMA is contraindicated in

   a. Unconscious patients

   b. Patients with an intact gag reflex

   c. Patients with an unstable neck injury

   d. Patients who cannot be positioned for tracheal intubation

124. Paralytic agents may **NOT** be used in the emergency intubation of

    a. Patients with facial hair

    b. Agitated trauma patients

    c. Combative patients

    d. Pediatric patients

125. All of the following are useful in RSI **except**

    a. Mallampati score

    b. Lidocaine

    c. Cricothyrotomy

    d. Preoxygenation

126. Air bags are most effective in

    a. Rear-impact collisions

    b. Frontal collisions

    c. Multiple collisions

    d. Rollover impacts

127. Which of the following statements regarding transport of a child in the ambulance is **FALSE**?

    a. Infants and young children can be transported in a child safety seat

    b. A child safety seat can be secured to a stretcher

    c. Older children can be secured to a stretcher

    d. The parent and child can be secured to a stretcher together

128. Hypovolemia may be associated with all of the following **except**

    a. Septic shock

    b. Hemorrhage

    c. Fainting

    d. Cardiogenic shock

129. Which of the following is a sign of uncompensated shock?

  a. Hypotension

  b. Unconsciousness

  c. Coma

  d. Combativeness

130. Jugular vein distention is associated with

  a. Anaphylactic shock

  b. Septic shock

  c. Cardiogenic shock

  d. Distributive shock

131. Which of the following wounds requires closure?

  a. Ring finger injury

  b. Abrasion from a motorcycle crash

  c. Contusion from a car accident

  d. Puncture wound from an animal bite

132. The wife of a 44-year-old man calls to report that her husband has suffered a deep wound to his forearm as the result of a broken power saw. On arrival, the wound is bleeding profusely. The first step in controlling hemorrhage should be to

  a. Apply a tourniquet

  b. Apply direct pressure

  c. Apply a splint

  d. Apply a pneumatic pressure device

133. Prehospital care of an open wound may involve all of the following **except**

    a. Applying antibacterial ointment

    b. Irrigating the wound with water

    c. Debridement of the wound

    d. Dressing the wound

134. After a building collapse, a construction worker is trapped beneath a steel beam for several hours. His right leg has been crushed under the beam and his left has been amputated. Initial treatment of this patient should include

    a. Aggressive hydration with 5% dextrose in water and 0.45% normal saline

    b. Fasciotomy of the right leg

    c. Administration of calcium chloride

    d. Administration of furosemide

135. Management of the patient's left leg should include

    a. Applying a tourniquet to the remaining portion of the left leg

    b. Searching for the amputated limb

    c. If found, treating the amputated limb in the same manner as avulsed tissue

    d. Fasciotomy to the remaining portion of the left leg

136. You are called to the scene of a car accident in which a 35-year-old man has hit a pole; damage to the vehicle is minimal, and no other cars were involved. The victim does not appear to be injured and claims he was not hurt; however, he admits to have been drinking before the accident and is clearly intoxicated. The MOI in this case is

    a. Positive

    b. Negative

    c. Uncertain

    d. Distraction

137. Which of the following statements regarding spinal injury is **FALSE**?

   a. Spinal injury can occur without SCI

   b. SCI only occurs with spinal injury

   c. SCI may occur without spinal injury

   d. SCI without spinal injury is more common in children

138. Which of the following statements regarding spinal immobilization is **FALSE**?

   a. A rigid cervical collar does not provide adequate spinal immobilization

   b. In immobilization to a long spine board, the torso should be immobilized before the head

   c. Short spine boards should be used for immobilization of patients in a confined space

   d. Short spine boards should be used for patients requiring immediate resuscitation

139. A 10-year-old boy has been ejected from an all-terrain recreational vehicle and has suffered potential spinal trauma. The boy is wearing a full-face helmet. Proper prehospital care for this patient should include all of the following **except**

   a. Removal of the helmet

   b. Manual in-line immobilization

   c. Immobilization on a short spine board

   d. Immobilization on a long spine board

140. A 45-year-old woman loses control of her vehicle on an icy road and rams into a tree. The patient complains that she has lost all feeling in her right leg and that she has "wet herself." Hypotension and vasodilation are present. This patient may be suffering from

a. Neurogenic hypotension

b. Spinal shock

c. Autonomic hyperreflexia

d. Spondylosis

141. Distended neck veins are usually associated with

a. Open pneumothorax

b. Closed pneumothorax

c. Tension pneumothorax

d. Flail chest

142. Which of the following statements regarding tension pneumothorax is **FALSE**?

a. Tension pneumothorax may result from sealing an open pneumothorax with occlusive dressing

b. Tension pneumothorax may be fatal

c. Tension pneumothorax may be relieved by thoracic decompression

d. Tension pneumothorax is primarily identified by chest percussion

143. Management of abdominal trauma should include all of the following **except**

a. Scene assessment

b. Fluid replacement

c. Replacement of eviscerated organs

d. Use of a PASG

144. Traction splints may be used for

    a. Pelvic fracture

    b. Hip injury

    c. Knee injury

    d. Femoral fracture

145. Which of the following statements regarding treatment of fractures and dislocations is **FALSE**?

    a. Knee realignment is indicated by a "popping" into the joint

    b. A dislocated elbow can be realigned at the scene

    c. Fractures and dislocated joints should be immobilized in the direction of injury

    d. Hip realignment is indicated by a "popping" into the joint

146. An extra heart sound may be indicative of

    a. Congestive heart failure

    b. Ventricular systole

    c. Ventricular diastole

    d. Myocardial infarction

147. The ECG lead aV$_F$ is an example of a

    a. Bipolar limb lead

    b. Unipolar limb lead

    c. Unipolar chest lead

    d. Bipolar chest lead

148. In an ECG reading, the QRS complex follows the

    a. Q-T interval

    b. T wave

    c. ST segment

    d. P wave

149. Which of the following methods may be used to calculate heart rate when the heart rhythm is irregular?

    a. Triplicate method

    b. Six-second count method

    c. R-R method

    d. Heart rate calculator ruler

150. All of the following may be used to treat paroxysmal supraventricular tachycardia **except**

    a. Adenosine

    b. Vagal maneuvers

    c. Magnesium

    d. Valsalva maneuver

Answers and Explanations

1. C. An anaphylactoid reaction is the most severe form of allergic reaction and is not mediated by an antigen-antibody reaction. A type I allergic reaction may lead to life-threatening anaphylaxis. Immunity can be natural or can be artificially induced through immunization.

2. D. Individuals in occupations that may involve prolonged exposure to latex, such as hairdressers, food handlers, healthcare workers, and tollbooth operators, are at high risk of latex allergy. Patients with asthma or with a genetic predisposition to allergies may also be at high risk; however, patients with allergic rhinitis are at no particular risk of latex allergy.

3. C. The first step in managing a patient with an anaphylactic reaction is to provide adequate airway support; the patient should be placed in a comfortable position and high-concentration oxygen should be administered. Intramuscular epinephrine may be given to patients with clinical signs of shock; however, intravenous epinephrine should only be given in rare instances and with authorization from medical direction. Saline is given only in the presence of hypotension or when the patient does not respond to epinephrine.

4. B. Beta-blockers can increase the severity of anaphylaxis and induce a severe reaction to epinephrine; however, beta agonists, antihistamines, corticosteroids, antiarrhythmics, and vasopressors may be given as additional drug therapy.

5. D. Signs of a mild allergic reaction include urticaria or hives, cramping or diarrhea, and bronchoconstriction; however, altered mental status, as indicated by a sense of impending doom, confusion, and agitation, is typically associated with anaphylaxis.

6. C. In performing defibrillation, paddles should not be placed over the sternum or over the generator of an implanted automatic defibrillator or pacemaker. Place one paddle to the right of the upper sternum below the clavicle and the other to the left of the left nipple immediately over the apex of the heart.

7. D. Various gels, creams, and pastes are useful in decreasing paddle-skin interface resistance; however, use only those made specifically for defibrillation and not for electrocardiogram monitoring. Pads soaked in saline are safe but those soaked in alcohol may ignite.

8. A. Nitroglycerin patches should be removed before defibrillation; placing paddles together can cause pitting, which may burn the patient. Alternating cardiopulmonary resuscitation with defibrillation may transfer gel from the patient's chest to the paddle handles. To remove an unwanted charge, simply turn off the defibrillator.

9. C. Asynchronous pacing is used less often than demand pacing, usually as only a last resort. Asynchronous pacing may be used in cases of asystole, to control tachydysrhythmia such as torsades de pointes, and in cases when artifact on the electrocardiogram interferes with its ability to read the actual heartbeat.

10. B. Transcutaneous cardiac pacing is primarily used in cases of symptomatic bradycardia, heart block associated with reduced cardiac output, or pacemaker failure. Cardiac pacing is usually ineffective in cardiac arrest or pulseless electrical activity and is not recommended in patients with open wounds or burns.

11. D. Resuscitation should not be attempted in patients with a valid Do Not Attempt Resuscitation (DNAR) order, in cases when vital functions have deteriorated, such as in patients with septic or cardiogenic shock, or in patients with asystole; however, resuscitation may be indicated in special cases, such as in young children

or in those with hypothermia, electrolyte abnormalities, toxin exposure, or drug overdose.

12. B. Initial defibrillation should be attempted at 360 J monophasic energy; initial defibrillation for pediatric patients is 2 J/kg, followed by 4 J/kg if necessary. Biphasic defibrillation of 115 J is as effective as monophasic defibrillation of 200 J; the optimal current for ventricular defibrillation is 30 to 40 A.

13. A. Patients with chronic obstructive pulmonary disease (COPD) typically have an acute episode of worsening dyspnea and may be leaning forward to aid breathing. These patients may use accessory muscles as well as pursed-lip breathing to aid in respiration.

14. C. The thin, barrel-chest appearance of this patient, as well as the presence of wheezing, rhonchi, and pursed-lip breathing, are indicative of emphysema.

15. C. Typical signs and symptoms of chronic bronchitis include chronic cyanosis, productive cough, and resistance on inspiration; pink or red complexion, nonproductive cough, and pursed-lip breathing are indicative of emphysema.

16. D. In all patients in respiratory distress, the paramedic should establish an IV line and apply a cardiac monitor. Pulse oximetry and administration of high-concentration oxygen are also indicated; however, oxygen should not be withheld to avoid reduction of the hypoxic drive.

17. B. In the acronym OPQRST, used in obtaining a focused history in patients with respiratory distress, O = onset, P = provocation, Q = quality, R = region and radiation, S = severity, and T = time.

18. C. Conditions indicative of a perfusion problem include shock, anemia, pulmonary embolism, and trauma; asthma is indicative of a ventilation problem and atherosclerosis and carbon dioxide poisoning of diffusion problems.

19. A. Patients with chronic bronchitis and emphysema, known together as chronic obstructive pulmonary disease (COPD), may have both COPD and asthma at the same time but in varying degrees of severity. Patients with emphysema are referred to as "pink puffers" due to increased production of red blood cells; those with bronchitis are referred to as "blue bloaters" because they often appear cyanotic. In contrast to adult-onset asthma, childhood asthma usually improves or resolves with age.

20. B. The primary goal in managing an acute asthma attack is to ensure an adequate airway and reverse the bronchospasm. After administering high-concentration oxygen and consulting medical direction, the next step is usually to administer a fast-acting bronchodilator such as albuterol. Continuous positive airway pressure (CPAP) and biphasic positive airway pressure (BiPAP) should only be used if the patient has adequate spontaneous respirations; ketamine is used to sedate a patient before endotracheal intubation.

21. C. Inspiratory wheezing may indicate the presence of secretions in the large airways but does not necessarily indicate upper airway occlusion.

22. C. Peak expiratory flow rate (PEFR) tests are used in patients experiencing an acute asthma attack to determine baseline airflow before drug administration. PEFR tests are not useful in children less than 5 years of age or in patients in severe respiratory distress. Positive end-expiratory pressure (PEEP) is often used in patients with adult respiratory distress syndrome (ARDS).

23. B. Initial management of a stroke patient should include providing life support, confirming signs and symptoms, and establishing the time of stroke onset to determine whether fibrinolytic therapy should be administered; the patient should then be transported to the hospital as soon as possible for definitive care. Management of hypertension is not indicated in the initial treatment of stroke.

24. D. Both the Cincinnati Prehospital Stroke Scale (CPSS) and the Los Angeles Prehospital Stroke Screen (LAPSS) are useful in diagnosing stroke; if the patient is conscious, obtaining a medical history may also be useful. 50% dextrose is administered during glucose analysis only when indicated.

25. C. Transient ischemic attacks (TIAs) present with the same signs and symptoms as those of stroke; thus, assessment of a patient with a TIA is the same as that for a patient with stroke. TIAs are important predictors of brain infarction; however, they are not associated with permanent neurological deficits.

26. A. The first step in treating a patient with abdominal pain is to survey the scene to determine whether the patient's condition is due to trauma or a medical condition; the area should be inspected for signs of alcohol or drug use, such as medication bottles. Pain medication should not be given to a patient with abdominal pain because it may mask critical signs and symptoms. Following the initial survey, a physical examination should be performed to identify any abdominal injuries. Transport should be provided only if abdominal pain persists for 6 or more hours.

27. D. In the mnemonic OPQRST, the letter P stands for provocative or palliative. The patient should be asked what improves or worsens pain; for example, whether sitting or lying down affects pain. The letter O stands for onset and S severity; past medical history is part of the SAMPLE history.

28. C. Pain location is included as part of the OPQRST evaluation (R or region); women of childbearing age should be asked about menstrual and/or pregnancy history. Changes in bowel habits and last meal or oral intake are key elements of the SAMPLE history in patients with abdominal pain.

29. A. Conditions associated with visceral or organ pain include cholecystitis, pancreatitis, and intestinal obstruction. Peritonitis and ulcer are associated with somatic pain, or constant pain localized to a specific area; morphine addiction is associated with dehydration, obstruction, and decreased intestinal motility.

30. B. Cholecystitis is often associated with cramping abdominal pain radiating to the upper right quadrant; pain increases in intensity, then subsides, and usually occurs at night, often after consuming fried or fatty foods. Cholecystitis is more common in women. Pancreatitis is associated with severe epigastric pain, often accompanied by abdominal distention; bowel obstruction usually results from fecal impaction or tumor. Crohn's disease is a chronic condition marked by diarrhea, anorexia, and weight loss.

31. C. Nasogastric intubation is indicated only in unusual circumstances and only under medical direction; nasogastric intubation is indicated in conscious patients with an intact gag reflex but may be attempted in unconscious patients with a protected airway. Complications associated with nasogastric intubation include gastrointestinal bleeding, nasal hemorrhage, and perforation of the esophagus.

32. A. Dialysis patients with chronic renal failure can tolerate increased potassium levels better than patients with normal kidney function; however, dialysis patients are at increased risk of hemorrhage and may suffer dysrhythmias resulting from myocardial ischemia. Peritoneal dialysis is slower than hemodialysis but is just as effective over time.

33. D. In the case of graft occlusion resulting from thrombus formation, attempting to clear the graft by irrigation or aspiration or obtaining blood pressure measurements in an extremity with an arteriovenous graft is not recommended; intravenous infusion of fluids should be initiated in an alternative site.

34. B. Gastric lavage should only be performed in patients who have ingested a lethal amount of poison within the last hour; in intubated or comatose patients, gastric lavage should be performed after tracheal intubation to prevent aspiration pneumonia. Gastric lavage can be safely performed in both adults and children.

35. C. Only normal saline should be used for gastric lavage in pediatric patients to prevent water absorption. Gastric lavage is contraindicated in the case of ingestion of low-viscosity hydrocarbons such as gasoline or caustic agents due to the increased risk of aspiration.

36. A. Syrup of ipecac is no longer the drug of choice in cases of poisoning and is not recommended for routine use; however, it is still commonly found in patients' homes. Syrup of ipecac is contraindicated in pregnant patients and in patients in a state of altered consciousness.

37. C. The antidote for calcium channel blocker ingestion is calcium; bicarbonate is indicated for cyclic antidepressants, ethanol for methanol, and glucagon for beta-blockers.

38. D. Baby oil is a hydrocarbon and ingestion is particularly dangerous; thus, the first step in treating hydrocarbon ingestion is to provide adequate ventilatory and circulatory support. Decontamination of the stomach or administration of activated charcoal or syrup of ipecac is not recommended for hydrocarbon ingestion.

39. B. Baby oil is a particularly dangerous hydrocarbon because of the risk of aspiration; asphalt, tar, and grease are not aspirated or absorbed in the gastrointestinal tract and thus do not have significant toxicity.

40. D. Ingestion of as little as 4 mL of methanol can cause blindness; cyanosis, hemolytic or aplastic anemia, and bacterial pneumonia are associated with hydrocarbon ingestion.

41. C. Ingestion of the marigold plant is not dangerous; however, ingestion of mistletoe, buttercups, or daffodils may be toxic.

42. A. Use of the cyanide antidote kit in patients with cyanide poisoning due to smoke inhalation may reduce the amount of hemoglobin needed for oxygen transport, resulting in anoxia and death. Inhalation of amyl nitrite followed by supplemental oxygen and administration of hydroxocobalamin may be useful in detoxification.

43. D. Removal of the tick with forceps, tweezers, or protected fingers is the principal treatment for tick bite; use of nail polish, isopropanol, or a burning match head are ineffective and may cause the tick to salivate or regurgitate into the bite wound.

44. C. Benzodiazepines are the primary treatment for cocaine overdose; alkalinization and anticonvulsant therapy may be useful in treating overdose of tricyclic antidepressants. Naloxone is effective in treating overdose of heroin and other opioids. Phencyclidine (PCP) overdose may result in violent or unpredictable behavior; thus, these patients are usually rapidly transported for physician evaluation.

45. B. Naloxone is indicated for treatment of overdose of opioids such as heroin, morphine, or codeine; diazepam may be used in treating cocaine, antipsychotic, or lysergic acid diethylamide (LSD) overdose.

46. A. Naloxone is used in treating opioid poisoning but is not indicated for treatment of meperidine-induced seizures; benzodiazepines may be used in the treatment of acute coronary and anticholinergic syndrome.

47. C. Electrical defibrillation or cardioversion may be used in treatment of drug-induced ventricular tachycardia or fibrillation. High-dose epinephrine and propranolol are contraindicated in sympathomimetic poisoning associated with refractory ventricular fibrillation; calcium is indicated in drug-induced cardiogenic shock.

48. B. The major mechanisms of heat loss are radiation, conduction, convection, and evaporation.

49. C. In a case of suspected heat stroke, the top priority following BLS and ALS measures is to initiate rapid cooling; however, submerging the patient in ice water or cold water can induce peripheral vasoconstriction and convulsions. The patient should be moved to a cool environment and his or her clothing should be removed; administration of too much fluid can result in pulmonary edema. Patients suffering from hypothermia should be covered with warm blankets and transported.

50. B. Sweating is usually absent in cases of heat stroke; changes in electrocardiogram and increased muscle tone are symptoms associated with hypothermia.

51. C. Active internal rewarming techniques, including peritoneal or pleural lavage, extracorporeal circulation, and use of esophageal warming tubes, are invasive and

are not recommended for out-of-hospital care. Replacing wet with dry clothing can help retain body heat; passive rewarming techniques, such as removing wet clothing and wrapping the patient in blankets, and active external rewarming through the use of radiant heat, forced hot air, or warmed IV fluids, are useful in managing hypothermia.

52. D. The most significant clinical factors in prehospital care of a drowning victim are duration of submersion and duration and severity of hypoxia. Aspiration of contaminants or amount of aspirated fluid do not affect outcome.

53. B. Henry's law, Dalton's law, and Boyle's law outline the properties of gases and are thus significant in pressure-related diving emergencies; Newton's law is relevant in the study of physics.

54. D. Acute mountain sickness can result in headache, anorexia, vomiting, and impaired memory; high-altitude pulmonary edema is characterized by cough with or without frothy sputum, and high-altitude cerebral edema may result in altered consciousness or coma.

55. C. According to the CDC guidelines regarding universal precautions for prevention of transmission of HIV, hepatitis B, or other blood-borne pathogens, exposure to vomitus in the absence of blood is not subject to universal precautions; however, universal precautions must apply to exposure to semen, vaginal secretions, tissue, and fluids such as synovial or amniotic fluid.

56. A. HCV is transmitted in the same manner as other forms of hepatitis and most often results from needle-stick injury; however, HCV is not often transmitted through sexual contact. Most patients with HCV infection are asymptomatic; no vaccine has yet been developed for HCV.

57. B. Tuberculosis (TB) should be suspected in HIV-positive patients with undiagnosed lung disease; typical signs and symptoms of TB include coughing, hemoptysis, fever, and fatigue. Pneumonia is an acute infection of the bronchioles and alveoli of the lungs marked by tachypnea, high-grade fever, and cough with yellow-green phlegm. Symptoms of hepatitis C virus (HCV) usually develop within 2 to 3 months of infection and include anorexia, nausea and vomiting, and generalized rashes; hepatitis B virus (HBV) is marked by an influenza-like illness that lasts less than 6 months and may lead to cirrhosis or other liver disease.

58. D. TB is most prevalent in homeless shelters, nursing homes, and other facilities and in patients with HIV infection. TB is most commonly transmitted by the coughing or sneezing of bacteria into the air and less often through the skin or mucous membranes.

59. A. A surgical mask is ineffective in preventing inhalation of TB bacteria; however, it should be placed on the patient before transport. NIOSH recommends use of an N-type respirator and an ambulance ventilation system including a high-efficiency particulate air (HEPA) filter to prevent paramedic exposure to TB while transporting the patient; a complete respiratory protection program should be implemented whenever respirators are required.

60. D. Nuchal rigidity, projectile vomiting, headache, and petechial rash are classic signs of meningitis. Tetanus is marked by stiffness of the jaw and rubella by a diffuse macular rash; measles is characterized by a blotchy red rash.

61. D. In treating a patient with signs and symptoms of meningitis, universal and body substance isolation (BSI) precautions should be taken, including placement of a surgical mask on the patient. Antibiotics are key in the treatment of meningitis and are usually given 30 to 60 minutes after arriving at the emergency department; analgesics are effective in the management of pneumonia.

62. B. Rabies vaccine is given by injection over a period of several weeks; however, injections are no longer given in the stomach. Tetanus prophylaxis may be indicated for treatment of the bite wound. If left untreated, rabies infection can result in eye and facial muscle paralysis. An animal suspected of being rabid should be killed by the proper authorities and examined for rabies antibodies.

63. A. More than 80% of severe acute respiratory syndrome (SARS) cases improve spontaneously; strict quarantine is the most effective mode of treatment. SARS is seldom transmitted via contact with family members or coworkers and is not transmitted through blood transfusion.

64. B. Bird flu is transmitted among birds and occasionally pigs but cannot be transmitted among humans; antiviral therapy is not indicated for bird flu prophylaxis due to reduce risk of developing a resistant strain of the virus.

65. D. Compressed air may allow infectious material to become airborne and should not be used to clean a vehicle or equipment used in transporting a severe acute respiratory syndrome (SARS) patient; used needles and scalpel blades should be collected in sharps containers and disposed of in accordance with hospital requirements and all non-patient areas of the vehicle should also be cleaned. Paramedics with suspected SARS exposure who are asymptomatic may continue working during the 10-day period following exposure.

66. C. In assessing a patient with a behavioral emergency, the first step should be to establish rapport by providing a limited and supportive interview; the paramedic should listen to the patient's account of events, showing support and empathy. The patient's personal space should be respected, and physical touch should be limited. Calling the police or using restraints is unnecessary if the patient is cooperative.

67. A. In managing a violent patient, the paramedic should offer him or her a final chance to cooperate before applying physical restraint; physical restraint is only warranted after all techniques to calm the patient have been exhausted. A single paramedic should not be left alone with a violent patient; at least four individuals should be present to help restrain the patient. If the patient is armed, the paramedic should move other individuals out of range, call law enforcement, then leave the scene. Chemical restraint should not be attempted without approval from medical direction.

68. C. Lithium is used in the treatment of bipolar disorder; diazepam is a benzodiazepine and haloperidol an antipsychotic used for chemical restraint. Diphenhydramine is used to reverse extrapyramidal side effects associated with antipsychotic drugs.

69. C. Before obtaining a patient history or examining the patient, the patient should be moved to a private area; obtaining a sexual history is irrelevant to patient care and may upset the patient. The patient's genitalia should be examined only if severe injury is suspected; the patient's clothing should be disturbed as little as possible to avoid damaging any evidence.

70. B. A pregnant trauma victim should be treated in the same manner as a nonpregnant victim; all pregnant women should be given high-concentration oxygen and transported. Transport should not be delayed to assess fetal heart rate. Women beyond 4 months' gestation should not be transported in the supine position to avoid hypotension; the left lateral recumbent position is preferred. The pneumatic antishock garment is rarely used and only under medical direction.

71. C. In managing a patient with third-trimester bleeding, vaginal examination may increase bleeding and/or induce labor and thus should not be attempted. Airway,

ventilatory, and circulatory support should be provided as needed and IV fluid therapy initiated; fundal height should be documented for baseline measurement.

72. A. The Apgar score (appearance, pulse, grimace, activity, respiration) should not be used to determine the need for resuscitation of a baby just born. Presence or absence of crying and/or breathing and appearance of muscle tone should be used to assess the infant; the amniotic fluid should be clear and without signs of infection.

73. B. Packing the vagina should not be attempted to control postpartum hemorrhage; oxytocin and uterine massage may aid in stimulating uterine contraction. Placing the infant close to the mother's breast facilitates breastfeeding and may promote uterine contraction.

74. D. Warning devices are generally used only during transport of patient with life- or limb-threatening injury; lights and sirens should never be used to provide absolute right of way. Police escorts may result in collision as a result of motorist confusion and should not be used in responding to a routine emergency call; low beams should be used during all responses regardless of weather conditions to increase visibility.

75. C. The 2-second rule is useful for gauging braking distance for conventional type I, II, or III emergency vehicles under normal road and weather conditions; braking distance should be increased for larger or heavier vehicles and under poor roadway or weather conditions.

76. D. Air ambulances have specific space and weight restrictions that may limit the number of patients, emergency and flight personnel, and equipment that can be carried. In the urban setting, ground ambulances are faster that air ambulances within a 30-mile range. Although fewer crashes occur with air than with ground ambulances, helicopter crashes have fewer survivors.

77. C. In this case, primary triage should be used to classify accident victims according to treatment priority; the only treatment given during primary triage is to ensure an airway or control severe hemorrhage.

78. B. The START, or simple triage and rapid treatment technique, is used to classify a patient's status in primary triage according to ability to walk, breathing, pulse/perfusion, and mental status; in secondary triage, the patient is reassessed and labeled with a tag indicating priority of care. Critical incident stress management is used to assist distressed rescue personnel after a large-scale incident.

79. A. According to the START technique of primary triage (simple triage and rapid treatment), patients who can walk and understand basic commands are classified as delayed or walking wounded; these patients should be advised to remain at the site for further assistance or to walk to another treatment site. If the patient is unable to walk, the respiratory rate should be assessed.

80. C. A patient with a carotid pulse but no radial pulse should be classified as critical; if both the carotid and radial pulses are present, mental status should be assessed before triage classification. Conscious patients who are able to walk are classified as delayed; if no pulse is present, the patient should be classified as dying.

81. A. Submerged victims should not be lifted onto a back board; rather, the board should be allowed to float up to the patient. Before attempting a water rescue, the paramedic should put on a personal flotation device (PFD); multiple victims submerged in the water should be directed to huddle together to conserve body heat, while a single victim should be told to assume the fetal or heat escape-lessening position (HELP).

82. C. Resuscitation should be attempted in all victims of prolonged exposure to extremely cold water unless death is obvious; rapid hypothermia can actually improve brain viability. Sudden exposure to extremely cold water can cause laryngospasm, resulting in aspiration, hypoxia, and unconsciousness. The effectiveness of the cold protective response depends on the patient's age, lung volume, position in the water, and water temperature.

83. B. On arrival at the site of a confined-space emergency, a copy of the Occupational Safety & Health Administration (OSHA) permit should be obtained to properly assess the scene; in the case of a cave-in or trench collapse, the paramedic should not approach the lip, as the risk of a second collapse is high. Shoring or a trench box is required for cave-ins 5 feet deep or greater; the self-contained breathing apparatus (SCBA) provides only a limited supply of air, may cause entrapment, or may have to be removed to reach the victim, and thus should not be used for confined-space rescue.

84. C. In the case of downed electrical wires, paramedics should not attempt to replace the wires or approach patients until the scene is safe; passengers inside a vehicle entrapped by downed wires should be directed to remain inside to avoid the risk of electrical injury.

85. B. In the case of both deployed and undeployed airbags, the 5-, 10-, 20 rule should be used to determine a safe distance during rescue: a distance of 5 inches should be used for side impact airbags, 10 inches for driver-side airbags, and 20 inches for passenger-side airbags. The car battery should be disconnected when a passenger is trapped behind an undeployed airbag; to verify that the battery has been disconnected, turn on the lights rather than the ignition. Do not place a hard board or other device between the passenger and the airbag.

86. C. During a rescue attempt, basic life support (BLS) techniques are mandatory, including airway control with supplemental oxygen. Advanced life support (ALS) techniques should only be provided if necessary; endotracheal intubation, IV lines, and ECG leads may complicate the rescue attempt.

87. C. In the case of a potentially violent situation, avoidance, tactical retreat, cover and concealment, and distraction and evasive maneuvers are useful tactics to ensure paramedic safety; confrontation should be avoided.

88. B. A bulletproof vest is effective against most handgun bullets and knives; however, it may not protect against thin or dual-edged weapons such as an ice pick.

89. A. The self-contained breathing apparatus (SCBA) provides the highest level of respiratory protection against hazardous materials; because an air-purifying respirator requires constant monitoring and must be fitted to the wearer, it is not recommended for protection against hazardous materials. Level C clothing is used for transport of contaminated patients; level D clothing provides only minimal protection.

90. D. Patient care in the hot zone should be limited to airway management, spinal immobilization, and hemorrhage control; removal of the patient from the hot zone is usually performed by trained personnel, such as firefighters and/or hazmat teams. IV therapy should only be given under the direction of a physician; invasive procedures such as wound debridement should not be performed to prevent hazardous materials from entering the patient's body.

91. B. Following a hazmat incident, the hazmat team will establish a decontamination corridor; rescue personnel should shower twice to remove any potential contaminants and should be debriefed as to the nature of the hazardous

substances, signs or symptoms of exposure, and any acute or chronic health issues that may arise.

92. C. Compared with adults, a child's liver and spleen are larger and more vascular and are thus more easily injured; children also have a larger body surface area-to-body mass ratio, increasing the risk of hypothermia, hyperthermia, and dehydration. Because children are able to use vasoconstriction to decrease the size of blood vessels, they are able to maintain blood pressure longer than adults; for this reason, a child in shock may have a normal blood pressure. In children, the muscles rather than the bones provide the primary means of support for the chest wall.

93. B. In assessing a child who is not acutely ill, the paramedic should allow the child to become more familiar with the paramedic team and medical equipment by conversing with the child and allowing him or her to play with the stethoscope; this "transition stage" may be helpful in putting the child at ease. In a seriously ill or injured child, vital signs should be monitored every 5 minutes and continuous electrocardiogram monitoring should be performed; the physical exam should be conducted from toe to head in children younger than 2 years and from head to toe in older children.

94. A. Barking cough, nasal flaring, cyanosis, and low-grade fever are indicative of croup; croup typically occurs in children 6 months to 4 years of age with a history of recent upper respiratory infection. Patients usually present at night with signs of respiratory distress and may be sitting upright to facilitate breathing. Croup is sometimes confused with epiglottitis, a bacterial infection in children 3 to 7 years of age characterized by swelling of the epiglottis and supraglottic structures; however, unlike croup, epiglottitis is of rapid onset and marked by high fever, drooling, and inspiratory stridor. Pneumonia is an acute infection of the lower airway and lungs marked by chest pain, rales, rhonchi, and tachypnea.

95. D. Symptoms of croup may be dramatically improved by exposure to cool humidified air; intubation and parenteral antibiotic therapy are indicated in a child with epiglottitis and bronchodilators in a child with severe pneumonia.

96. C. Intubation is usually not indicated in children with status epilepticus unless the child does not respond to initial treatment. Diazepam is effective in treating seizures in the majority of cases; glucagon may be used to treat hypoglycemia. Cardiac monitoring is used to detect cardiac rhythm or conduction abnormalities.

97. B. Insulin is usually not given in the prehospital setting in a child with suspected hyperglycemia; glucose testing should be performed following airway, ventilatory, and circulatory support. IV fluid therapy may be given if the child is dehydrated; if hyperglycemia cannot be confirmed with glucose testing, dextrose may be given to rule out hypoglycemia.

98. D. Possible causes of sudden infant death syndrome (SIDS) include immaturity of the central nervous system, upper airway obstruction, brainstem abnormalities, and cardiac conduction disorders; suffocation, regurgitation or aspiration of vomitus, and allergies are not associated with SIDS.

99. B. The presence of sudden tachycardia and tachypnea, as well as mild discomfort and edema of the calf, is indicative of pulmonary embolism; in the elderly, pulmonary embolism may be associated with congestive heart failure (CHF). Because the signs and symptoms of pulmonary embolism are similar to those of bacterial pneumonia, the two conditions are often mistaken for each other. Dyspnea is commonly seen in elderly patients with bacterial pneumonia, pulmonary embolism, myocardial infarction, and other conditions, making diagnosis difficult. Signs and symptoms of heart failure include dry, hacking productive cough, nocturia, and anorexia.

100. A. Aggressive airway management is indicated in chronic obstructive pulmonary disease (COPD) to treat acidosis and hypoxia, which may be life-threatening. Emergency care for patients with pulmonary embolism and bacterial pneumonia should provide adequate airway, ventilatory, and circulatory support; in patients with cerebral vascular disease, the primary goal of treatment is to identify stroke and transport the patient for immediate care.

101. C. Delirium is characterized by rapid onset of disorientation to time and place and may result from physical illness; dementia and Alzheimer's disease are marked by slow, progressive loss of awareness.

102. B. Rapid fluid IV administration may cause volume overload in the elderly; thus, the paramedic must be careful not to overhydrate an older patient. Partial pressure of oxygen in arterial blood (PaO_2) decreases with age; elderly patients may require higher arterial pressures for perfusion of vital organs as a result of atherosclerotic peripheral vascular disease. Adjustment of heart rate and stroke volume may be decreased in the elderly in response to hypovolemia.

103. D. The rule of nines is used to estimate burn injury size for adults and children over 10 years of age; it may be difficult to apply to irregularly shaped burns or burns scattered over a large area of the body.

104. B. Moderate burns may be classified as partial-thickness burns covering 15% to 25% of body surface area (BSA) in adults and 10% to 20% of BSA in children or the elderly and full-thickness burns covering less than 10% of BSA; burns from contact with caustic chemicals or high-voltage electricity may be classified as major burns.

105. C. Covering the patient with a sterile blanket will preserve body heat and prevent too much heat loss. Applying ointment or ice to a burn may increase the

severity of the injury and/or cause shock. Removal of blisters is at the discretion of the hospital burn-unit and not the concern of the paramedic.

106. B. In patients with carbon monoxide poisoning, the proper line of treatment is to ensure a patent airway, provide ventilation, and administer high-concentration oxygen; sodium thiosulfate and hyperbaric oxygen may also be given. The pulse oximeter is not a reliable indicator of effective oxygenation in cases of carbon monoxide poisoning.

107. C. Contrary to popular belief, asking a patient directly about his or her suicidal intentions does not encourage the patient to commit suicide; following medical care, establishing rapport with the patient and providing emotional support are essential. Law enforcement should only be consulted when the patient is armed.

108. A. A carbon monoxide level of 10% is commonly seen in smokers, truck drivers, traffic police, and others who are chronically exposed to carbon monoxide and is asymptomatic. A carbon monoxide level of 20% may cause nausea and vomiting, 30% may cause electrocardiogram abnormalities, and 40% to 60% may cause coma.

109. D. Administering osmotic diuretics and/or steroids to a patient with increasing intracranial pressure may reduce cerebral edema and inflammation. IV fluid therapy should be restricted in such patients; the Valsalva maneuver may increase intraabdominal pressure. Blood replacement therapy is used in patients with acute blood loss.

110. B. Pulmonary capillary wedge pressure (PCWP), pulmonary artery pressure (PAP) monitoring, and left atrial pressure (LAP) monitoring provide an accurate measure of left ventricular function; right atrial pressure (RAP) monitoring directly measures pressure in the right atrium and indirectly measures right ventricular pressure.

111. C. Epinephrine stimulates respiration and ventilation. Diazepam and morphine may decrease respiration; however, aspirin does not significantly affect respiratory function.

112. A. Morphine is considered a Pregnancy Category B drug and may be given to a pregnant woman in low doses for a short period of time; aspirin and diazepam are Category D drugs and should not be given during pregnancy except in the case of life-threatening disease. Oxytocin is administered after delivery to control postpartum bleeding.

113. C. Category C drugs may be given in pregnancy only if the potential benefit justifies the fetal risk; Category X drugs carry significant fetal risk and are contraindicated in pregnancy. Category B drugs have not been confirmed to provide a risk to pregnant women; Category D drugs are only indicated in the case of life-threatening disease.

114. B. The nasal cannula delivers only low-concentration oxygen and thus should be reserved for patients with chest pain or chronic pulmonary disease; it should not be used in patients with severe hypoxia, apnea, or respiratory insufficiency.

115. A. The bag-mask device may be used in patients with respiratory insufficiency or with a variety of pathological conditions; the nasal cannula and partial nonbreather and nonbreather masks should not be used in patients with apnea or respiratory insufficiency.

116. B. Use of the oropharyngeal or nasopharyngeal airway is indicated in an unconscious patient; the jaw-thrust position without the head-tilt technique should be used in those with suspected spinal injury. In the mouth-to-nose technique, the paramedic should keep one hand on the patient's forehead and use the other to close the patient's mouth. The mouth-to-stoma ventilation method is bacteriologically safer than the mouth-to-mouth technique.

117. A. The bag-mask device is primarily used for pediatric patients in respiratory arrest and should not be used to provide supplemental oxygen to a spontaneously breathing child; it may be used with a mask in patients who have not been intubated and is effective in extreme environmental temperatures.

118. D. The nasal airway may be used in unconscious patients and in those with cervical spine injury or seizures; however, it is contraindicated in patients with fractures of the basal skull or facial bones.

119. B. Cuffed endotracheal tubes are not indicated for infants or children under 8 years of age because narrowing of the cricoid cartilage acts as a natural cuff and prevents air leakage; they may, however, be used in older children.

120. D. Blind intubation is not an accepted prehospital procedure and should only be performed when the airway cannot be visualized due to the presence of blood or other secretions, in the case of patient entrapment, or in disaster situations with many victims and limited equipment. Nasotracheal intubation is a blind procedure and is only indicated in patients with spontaneous respirations, when laryngoscopy cannot be performed, or when movement of the cervical spine is limited; blind intubation is not indicated in patients with spinal injury.

121. C. Inaccurate pulse oximeter readings may result from a variety of factors, including hypotension, jaundice, hypothermia/vasoconstriction, and patient use of nail polish.

122. D. Manual in-line stabilization is required for intubation of patients with suspected spinal injuries; intubation of these patients is dangerous and must be authorized by medical direction.

123. B. The laryngeal mask airway (LMA) may be used in patients with an unstable neck injury, when conventional endotracheal intubation is unsuccessful, or when the patient cannot be positioned for tracheal intubation; patients must be unresponsive and without an intact gag reflex.

124. A. Paralytic agents are indicated in agitated or combative patients who require emergency intubation, such as those with a head injury or other trauma, and are acceptable for use in children; however, these agents should not be used in patients in whom ventilation or intubation may be difficult, such as those with facial hair, short necks, or obstructions.

125. C. Rapid sequence intubation (RSI) is used to rapidly bring a patient to an unconscious state through complete neuromuscular paralysis. The Mallampati score is used to assess the difficulty of intubation; preoxygenation with 100% oxygen is then accomplished, followed by pretreatment with lidocaine to prevent an increase in intracranial pressure and/or laryngospasm. Cricothyrotomy should only be performed if RSI is unsuccessful.

126. B. Airbags are most effective in frontal or near-frontal collisions.

127. D. A parent and child should never be secured to a stretcher together; however, a child safety seat can be safely secured to a stretcher using two belts placed at a 90º angle to each other. Infants and young children can be transported safely in a conventional child safety seat; older children can be secured to a stretcher.

128. C. Hypovolemia is associated with a variety of conditions and injuries such as hemorrhage, dehydration, burns, endocrine disorders, and tissue injury. Hypovolemia may occur in septic shock, and elements of cardiogenic shock may

occur in hypovolemia; fainting is associated with vasogenic shock, a mild, reversible form of shock.

129. B. Unconsciousness, delayed capillary refill, and decreased systolic and diastolic blood pressure are signs of uncompensated shock. Hypotension and coma are signs of irreversible shock; patients in compensated shock may be confused or combative.

130. C. Patients in cardiogenic shock may show signs of congestive heart failure such as jugular vein distention. Anaphylactic shock and septic shock are types of distributive shock, which may result from vasodilation; signs of distributive shock include warm, flushed skin.

131. A. Wounds that require closure include ring finger injuries, wounds to the face, lips, or eyebrows, wounds over joints, and degloving injuries; abrasions are partial-thickness skin injuries resulting from the scraping or rubbing away of layers of skin. Contusions result from blood vessel disruption below the epidermis and may cause bruising; puncture wounds such as those caused by an animal bite are generally small but may result in severe injury to underlying tissue.

132. B. The first step in controlling hemorrhage should be to apply direct pressure over the injury; a pressure dressing may then be applied over the wound and secured with an elastic bandage. Splinting alone is not effective as a means to control bleeding; a pneumatic pressure device should be used only after other methods have been tried to control bleeding. A tourniquet is not indicated as a means to control hemorrhage and should be used only as a last resort.

133. C. Prehospital care of an open wound usually involves cleansing the wound with sterile water, applying an antibacterial ointment if the patient is not allergic, and dressing the wound; debridement of the wound should not be attempted.

134. A. Crush syndrome may result from prolonged immobilization or compression such as in a building collapse or other catastrophic event when patient rescue has been delayed for several hours. Treatment of potential crush syndrome should include administration of high concentration oxygen, aggressive hydration with 5% dextrose in water and 0.45% normal saline, and alkalinization of the urine; calcium chloride is not indicated unless the patient is at risk of hyperkalemia. Furosemide may acidify the urine and should not be given; fasciotomy of a crushed limb is not recommended in the prehospital setting because of the risk of infection and must be authorized by medical direction.

135. C. Transport should not be delayed to search for an amputated limb; however, if the amputated limb is found, it should be treated in the same manner as avulsed tissue. Direct pressure and elevation should be used to control hemorrhage the remaining portion of the left leg; fasciotomy or application of a tourniquet is not recommended.

136. C. The mechanism of injury (MOI) must be assessed to determine the need for spinal immobilization. Spinal immobilization is necessary in the case of a positive MOI, such as a high-speed motor vehicle accident, a fall from greater than 3 times the patient's height, or a blunt or penetrating injury near the patient's spine, but is not required when the MOI is negative, as in the case of a twisted ankle, an object dropped on the foot, or an isolated soft-tissue injury. When the MOI is uncertain, as in the case of a low-speed motor vehicle crash, the paramedic must assess the reliability of the patient to determine the need for spinal immobilization; patients who are intoxicated, in an abnormal mental state, or who have distracting injuries are not considered reliable.

137. B. Spinal injury can occur with or without spinal cord injury (SCI); likewise, SCI can occur without spinal injury. SCI without radiological evidence of spinal injury is more commonly seen in children.

138. D. Short spine boards are primarily used for spinal immobilization of patients in a sitting position or in a confined space; a rigid collar alone is insufficient for spinal immobilization and should be used in conjunction with a short or long spine board. Long spine boards should be used for spinal immobilization of unstable patients with life-threatening injuries, patients requiring immediate resuscitation, or in situations where the time required to apply the device would put the patient's life in jeopardy. Immobilization of the torso to a long spine board should be performed before immobilizing the head.

139. C. A short spine board should be used for patients in a sitting position or in a confined space. Prehospital care of a pediatric patient with suspected spinal injury should include manual in-line immobilization, placement of a rigid cervical collar, and immobilization on a long spine board; an adult long spine board may be used if a pediatric device is not available. Full-face helmets should be removed to assess the patient's airway and ventilatory function.

140. B. Signs and symptoms of spinal shock include paralysis distal to the injury site, hypotension, vasodilation, and loss of bowel and bladder control; neurogenic hypotension is a rare condition and is not usually a cause of hypotension in patients with suspected spine injury. Autonomic hyperreflexia is marked by paroxysmal hypertension, bradycardia, and distended bladder or rectum; spondylosis is a structural defect of the spine and may result in stress fracture.

141. C. Tension pneumothorax is a life-threatening condition and must be managed immediately in the prehospital setting; signs and symptoms of tension pneumothorax include distended neck veins, diminished or absent breath sounds, increasing dyspnea, and hypotension. Open pneumothorax results from exposure of the pleural space to atmospheric pressure due to chest injury and is characterized by a sucking or gurgling sound through the open chest wound; closed pneumothorax occurs in patients with penetrating chest trauma and is marked by

chest pain, dyspnea, and tachypnea. Flail chest occurs when three or more ribs are fractured in two or more places and is characterized by paradoxical movement of the injured section of the chest wall during breathing.

142. D. Tension pneumothorax is an often fatal condition that occurs when air in the thoracic cavity is trapped in the pleural space; the condition may result from sealing an open pneumothorax with an occlusive dressing. Chest percussion alone is not reliable in identifying tension pneumothorax; thoracic decompression may be used to relieve tension pneumothorax in patients with closed chest trauma.

143. C. Management of an abdominal injury should be limited to stabilizing the patient and rapidly transporting him or her for surgical care; eviscerated organs should not be replaced into the peritoneal cavity because of the risk of infection. A thorough on-scene survey should be performed to identify the cause of the abdominal injury; airway maintenance, ventilatory support, and fluid replacement should be provided, and use of a pneumatic antishock garment (PASG) may be indicated depending on local protocol.

144. D. Traction splints should be used only for midshaft femoral fractures and should not be used for injuries of the hip or knee or fractures of the pelvis.

145. B. A severe fracture or dislocated joint (with exception of elbow) can be safely realigned and should be immobilized in the direction of the injury; successful realignment of the knee or hip is indicated by a "popping" into the joint. Realignment of a dislocated elbow should never be attempted in the prehospital setting.

146. A. An extra heart sound may be heard before S_1 or after S_2 and may be indicative of congestive heart failure. The first heart sign occurs during ventricular

systole and the second during ventricular diastole; heart sounds are not indicative of myocardial infarction.

147. B. The augmented limb lead aV_F is an example of a unipolar electrocardiogram (ECG) lead; limb leads I, II, and II are bipolar limb leads and V_1 to V_6 unipolar chest leads.

148. D. The QRS complex follows the P wave; the ST segment immediately follows the QRS complex. The T wave is the first deviation from the ST segment and ends with the return of the T wave to baseline. The Q-T interval is measured from the beginning of the QRS complex to the end of the T wave.

149. B. The triplicate and R-R methods are useful in determining heart rate only when the heart rhythm is regular; when used alone, the heart rate calculator ruler is not a reliable method of calculating heart rate and is accurate only when the rhythm is regular. Although the 6-second count method is the least accurate means of determining heart rate, it is useful in estimating heart rate in the presence of an irregular rhythm.

150. C. Vagal maneuvers and adenosine should be used as first-line treatment of paroxysmal supraventricular tachycardia; the Valsalva maneuver may successfully terminate tachycardia. Magnesium is used in the treatment of atrial fibrillation or flutter.

Special Report: Which Study Guides and Practice Tests Are Worth Your Time

We believe the following practice tests and guide present uncommon value to our customers who wish to "really study" for the EMT-P tests. While our manual teaches some valuable tricks and tips that no one else covers, learning the basic coursework tested on the exam is also necessary.

Practice Tests

Practice Test Questions

http://www.rescuehouse.com/quizzes/emsquizzes.php

Study Guides

EMT-Paramedic (P) PreTest Self Assessment and Review

http://www.amazon.com/exec/obidos/tg/detail/-/0071341560/qid=1083611447/sr=8-8/ref=sr_8_xs_ap_i8_xgl14/103-0364440-8271065?v=glance&s=books&n=507846

Paramedic Exam 2E

http://www.amazon.com/exec/obidos/tg/detail/-/1576853551/qid=1083611571/sr=8-4/ref=sr_8_xs_ap_i4_xgl14/103-0364440-8271065?v=glance&s=books&n=507846

Flashcards

EMT Flashcards

http://www.flashcardsecrets.com/emt

Special Report: Difficult Clients

Every EMT will eventually get a difficult client on their list of responsibilities. These individuals can be mentally, physically, and emotionally combative in many different environments. Consequently, care of these persons should be conducted in a manner for personal and self-protection of the EMT. Some of the key guidelines are as follows:

1. Never allow yourself to be cornered in a room with an individual positioned between you and the door.
2. Don't escalate the tension with verbal bantering. Basically, don't argue with the individual.
3. Ask permission before performing any normal tasks in an individual's environment whenever possible.
4. Discuss your concerns with other people on the scene. Consult the acting supervisor if necessary, especially when safety is an issue.
5. Get help from other individuals when offering care. Get a witness if you are anticipating abuse of any kind.
6. Remove yourself from the situation if you are concerned about your personal safety at all times.
7. If attacked, defend yourself with the force necessary for self-protection and attempt to separate from the individual.
8. Don't put yourself in a position to be hurt.
9. Get the necessary help for all transfers.
10. Respect the individual's personal property.
11. Get assistance quickly, via vocal projection or the radio, if a situation becomes violent or abusive.
12. Fill out an incident report for proper documentation of the occurrence.

Special Report: Guidelines for Standard Precautions

Standard precautions are precautions taken to avoid contracting various diseases and preventing the spread of disease to those who have compromised immunity. Some of these diseases include human immunodeficiency virus (HIV), acquired immunodeficiency syndrome (AIDS), and hepatitis B (HBV). Standard precautions are needed since many diseases do not display signs or symptoms in their early stages. Standard precautions mean to treat all body fluids/ substances as if they were contaminated. These body fluids include but are not limited to the following blood, semen, vaginal secretions, breast milk, amniotic fluid, feces, urine, peritoneal fluid, synovial fluid, cerebrospinal fluid, secretions from the nasal and oral cavities, and lacrimal and sweat gland excretions. This means that standard precautions should be used with all patients.

1. A shield for the eyes and face must be used if there is a possibility of splashes from blood and body fluids.
2. If possibility of blood or body fluids being splashed on clothing, you must wear a plastic apron.
3. Gloves must be worn if you could possibly come in contact with blood or body fluids. They are also needed if you are going to touch something that may have come in contact with blood or body fluids.
4. Hands must be washed even if you were wearing gloves. Hands must be washed and gloves must be changed between patients. Wash hands with at a dime size amount of soap and warm water for about 30 seconds. Singing "Mary had a little lamb" is approximately 30 seconds.
5. Blood and body fluid spills must be cleansed and disinfected using a solution of one part bleach to 10 parts water.

6. Used needles must be separated from clean needles. Throw both the needle and the syringe away in the sharps' container. The sharps' container is made of puncture proof material.

Special precautions must be taken to dispose of biomedical waste. Biomedical waste includes but is not limited to the following: laboratory waste, pathology waste, liquid waste from suction, all sharp object, bladder catheters, chest tubes, IV tubes, and drainage containers. Biomedical waste is removed from a by trained personal.

The health care professional is legally and ethically responsible for adhering to standard precautions. They may prevent you from contracting a fatal disease or from a patient contracting a disease from you that could be deadly.

Special Report: Basic Review of Types of Fractures

A fracture is defined as a break in a bone that may sometimes involve cartilaginous structures. A fracture can be classified according to its cause or the type of break. The following definitions are used to describe breaks.

1. Traumatic fracture – break in a bone resulting from injury
2. Spontaneous fracture – break in a bone resulting from disease
3. Pathologic fracture – another name for a spontaneous fracture
4. Compound fracture – occurs when fracture bone is exposed to the outside by an opening in the skin
5. Simple fracture - occurs when a break is contained within the skin
6. Greenstick fracture - a traumatic break that is incomplete and occurs on the convex surface of the bend in the bone
7. Fissured fracture – a traumatic break that involves an incomplete longitudinal break
8. Comminuted fracture – a traumatic break that involves a complete fracture that results in several bony fragments
9. Transverse fracture – a traumatic break that is complete and occurs at a right angle to the axis of the bone
10. Oblique fracture- a traumatic break that occurs at an angle other than a right angel to the axis of the bone.
11. Spiral fracture – a traumatic break that occurs by twisting a bone with extreme force

A compound fracture is much more dangerous than a simple break. This is due to the break in skin that can allow microorganisms to infect the injured tissue. When a fracture occurs, blood vessels within the bone and its periosteum are disrupted.

The periosteum, covering of fibrous connective tissue on the surface of the bone, may also be damaged or torn.

Special Report: High Frequency Terms

The following terms were compiled as high frequency EMT test terms. I recommend printing out this list and identifying the terms you are unfamiliar with. Then, use a medical dictionary or the internet to look up the terms you have questions about. Take one section per day if you have the time to maximize recall.

A

Acquired immunodeficiency syndrome

Amenorrhea

Aneurysm

Angina pectoris

Angiogenesis

Anklyosing spondylitis

Anxiety

Appendicitis

Arterial disease

Arteriosclerosis

Arthralgia

Arthritis

Atypical angina

B

Back pain

Blood cultures

Bradycardia

Braxton-Hicks contractions

Bronchiectasis

Bulimia

C

CAD

Cancer

Candidiasis

Cardiac disease

Carpal tunnel syndrome

Chest pain

Chest x-ray

Cirrhosis

COLD

Corticosteroids

D

Degenerative heart disease

Diabetes insipidus

Diabetes mellitus

Diabetic nephropathy

Dialysis

Diaphoresis

Down's syndrome

DVT

Dyspnea

E

Ectopic pregnancy

Electrocardiogram (ECG)

Embolism

Emphysema

Endocrine system

Epinephrine

Esophagitis

F

Fallopian tube

Fatigue

Fecal incontinence

Fibrillation

Fibromyalgia syndrome

G

Gangrene

Glucagon

Glucose tolerance test

Guillai-Barre' syndrome

H

Heart failure

Heart rate

Hemophilia

Hemorrhage

Heparin

Hepatitis (A-E)

Herpes zoster

Hiatal hernia

HIV

Hyponatremia

Hypothyroidism

Hypoxia

Hysterectomy

I

Immune serum globulin

Induration

Inflammatory bowel disease

Inhibitors

Interferon

Ischemic Heart Disease

J

Jaundice

Joint pain

Joint sepsis

Jevenile rheumatoid arthritis

K

Kidney failure

Kidney stones

L

Labile hypertension

Lactation

Low back pain

Lymphocyctes

M

Macrophages

Menarche

Ménière's disease

Metabolism

Multiple sclerosis

Myalgias

N

Neck pain

Neomycin

Night sweats

Nitrates

Nitroglycerin

Nocturnal angina

Norepinephrine

Nystagmus

O

Orthostatic hypotension

Osteoarthritis

Osteoporosis

P

Pain–joint

Palmar erythema

Palpitations

Pancreatitis

Parathyroid hormone

Paresthesia

Parkinson's disease

Pelvic inflammatory disease (PID)

Pericarditis

Pregnancy

Psychological support

Pulmonary edema

Q

Quadriceps

R

RA- Rheumatoid arthritis

Referred pain

Renal failure

Respiration

Rheumatic fever

Right ventricular failure

S

Sciatica

Scleroderma

Serotonin

Serum cholesterol

Sex hormones

Shoulder pain

Sickle cell anemia

Sinus bradycardia

Sinus tachycardia

Smoking

Systolic rate

T

Tendinitis

Thyroid gland

Tissue necrosis

Trauma

Tuberculosis

U

Ulceration

Umbilical pain

Ureter obstruction

Urethritis

Urinary bladder

Urinary tract infection

V

Vaginal bleeding

Vaginal lubricant

Ventricular failure

Vertigo

Vital signs

Vomiting

W

Weight gain

CPR Review/Cheat Sheet

Topic	New Guidelines
Conscious Choking	5 back blows, then 5 abdominal thrusts- adult/child
Unconscious Choking	5 chest compressions, look, 2 breaths-adult/child/infant
Rescue Breaths	Normal Breath given over 1 second until chest rises
Chest Compressions to Ventilation Ratios (Single Rescuer)	30:2 – Adult/Child/Infant
Chest Compressions to Ventilation Ratios (Two Rescuer)	30:2 – Adult 15:2 – Child/Infant
Chest Compression rate	About 100/minute – Adult/Child/Infant
Chest Compression Land marking Method	Simplified approach – center of the chest – Adult/Child 2 or 3 fingers, just below the nipple line at the center of the chest - Infant
AED	1 shock, then 2 minutes (or 5 cycles) of CPR
Anaphylaxis	Assist person with use of prescribed auto injector
Asthma	Assist person with use of prescribed inhaler

- Check the scene
- Check for responsiveness – ask, "Are you OK?"
- Adult - call 911, then administer CPR
- Child/Infant – administer CPR for 5 cycles, then call 911
- Open victim's airway and check for breathing – look, listen, and feel for 5 - 10 seconds
- Two rescue breaths should be given, 1 second each, and should produce a visible chest rise
- If the air does not go in, reposition and try 2 breaths again
- Check victim's pulse – chest compressions are recommended if an infant or child has a rate less than 60 per minute with signs of poor perfusion.
- Begin 30 compressions to 2 breaths at a rate of 1 breath every 5 seconds for Adult; 1 breath every 3 seconds for child/infant
- Continue 30:2 ratio until victim moves, AED is brought to the scene, or professional help arrives

Aed

- ADULT/ Child over 8 years old - use Adult pads
- Child 1-8 years old – use Child pads or use Adult pads by placing one on the chest and one on the back of the child
- Infant under 1 year of age - AED not recommended

Secret Key #1 - Time is Your Greatest Enemy

Pace Yourself

Wear a watch. At the beginning of the test, check the time (or start a chronometer on your watch to count the minutes), and check the time after every few questions to make sure you are "on schedule."

If you are forced to speed up, do it efficiently. Usually one or more answer choices can be eliminated without too much difficulty. Above all, don't panic. Don't speed up and just begin guessing at random choices. By pacing yourself, and continually monitoring your progress against your watch, you will always know exactly how far ahead or behind you are with your available time. If you find that you are one minute behind on the test, don't skip one question without spending any time on it, just to catch back up. Take 15 fewer seconds on the next four questions, and after four questions you'll have caught back up. Once you catch back up, you can continue working each problem at your normal pace.

Furthermore, don't dwell on the problems that you were rushed on. If a problem was taking up too much time and you made a hurried guess, it must be difficult. The difficult questions are the ones you are most likely to miss anyway, so it isn't a big loss. It is better to end with more time than you need than to run out of time.

Lastly, sometimes it is beneficial to slow down if you are constantly getting ahead of time. You are always more likely to catch a careless mistake by working more slowly than quickly, and among very high-scoring test takers (those who are likely to have lots of time left over), careless errors affect the score more than mastery of material.

Secret Key #2 - Guessing is not Guesswork

You probably know that guessing is a good idea - unlike other standardized tests, there is no penalty for getting a wrong answer. Even if you have no idea about a question, you still have a 20-25% chance of getting it right.

Most test takers do not understand the impact that proper guessing can have on their score. Unless you score extremely high, guessing will significantly contribute to your final score.

Monkeys Take the Test

What most test takers don't realize is that to insure that 20-25% chance, you have to guess randomly. If you put 20 monkeys in a room to take this test, assuming they answered once per question and behaved themselves, on average they would get 20-25% of the questions correct. Put 20 test takers in the room, and the average will be much lower among guessed questions. Why?

1. The test writers intentionally writes deceptive answer choices that "look" right. A test taker has no idea about a question, so picks the "best looking" answer, which is often wrong. The monkey has no idea what looks good and what doesn't, so will consistently be lucky about 20-25% of the time.

2. Test takers will eliminate answer choices from the guessing pool based on a hunch or intuition. Simple but correct answers often get excluded, leaving a 0% chance of being correct. The monkey has no clue, and often gets lucky with the best choice.

This is why the process of elimination endorsed by most test courses is flawed and detrimental to your performance- test takers don't guess, they make an ignorant stab in the dark that is usually worse than random.

$5 Challenge

Let me introduce one of the most valuable ideas of this course- the $5 challenge:

You only mark your "best guess" if you are willing to bet $5 on it.

You only eliminate choices from guessing if you are willing to bet $5 on it.

Why $5? Five dollars is an amount of money that is small yet not insignificant, and can really add up fast (20 questions could cost you $100). Likewise, each answer choice on one question of the test will have a small impact on your overall score, but it can really add up to a lot of points in the end.

The process of elimination IS valuable. The following shows your chance of guessing it right:

If you eliminate wrong answer choices until only this many answer choices remain:	1	2	3
Chance of getting it correct:	100%	50%	33%

However, if you accidentally eliminate the right answer or go on a hunch for an incorrect answer, your chances drop dramatically: to 0%. By guessing among all the answer choices, you are GUARANTEED to have a shot at the right answer.

That's why the $5 test is so valuable- if you give up the advantage and safety of a pure guess, it had better be worth the risk.

What we still haven't covered is how to be sure that whatever guess you make is truly random. Here's the easiest way:

Always pick the first answer choice among those remaining.

Such a technique means that you have decided, **before you see a single test question**, exactly how you are going to guess- and since the order of choices tells you nothing about which one is correct, this guessing technique is perfectly random.

This section is not meant to scare you away from making educated guesses or eliminating choices- you just need to define when a choice is worth eliminating. The $5 test, along with a pre-defined random guessing strategy, is the best way to make sure you reap all of the benefits of guessing.

Secret Key #3 - Practice Smarter, Not Harder

Many test takers delay the test preparation process because they dread the awful amounts of practice time they think necessary to succeed on the test. We have refined an effective method that will take you only a fraction of the time.

There are a number of "obstacles" in your way to succeed. Among these are answering questions, finishing in time, and mastering test-taking strategies. All must be executed on the day of the test at peak performance, or your score will suffer. The test is a mental marathon that has a large impact on your future.

Just like a marathon runner, it is important to work your way up to the full challenge. So first you just worry about questions, and then time, and finally strategy:

Success Strategy

1. Find a good source for practice tests.
2. If you are willing to make a larger time investment, consider using more than one study guide- often the different approaches of multiple authors will help

you "get" difficult concepts.

3. Take a practice test with no time constraints, with all study helps "open book." Take your time with questions and focus on applying strategies.

4. Take a practice test with time constraints, with all guides "open book."

5. Take a final practice test with no open material and time limits

If you have time to take more practice tests, just repeat step 5. By gradually exposing yourself to the full rigors of the test environment, you will condition your mind to the stress of test day and maximize your success.

Secret Key #4 - Prepare, Don't Procrastinate

Let me state an obvious fact: if you take the test three times, you will get three different scores. This is due to the way you feel on test day, the level of preparedness you have, and, despite the test writers' claims to the contrary, some tests WILL be easier for you than others.

Since your future depends so much on your score, you should maximize your chances of success. In order to maximize the likelihood of success, you've got to prepare in advance. This means taking practice tests and spending time learning the information and test taking strategies you will need to succeed.

Never take the test as a "practice" test, expecting that you can just take it again if you need to. Feel free to take sample tests on your own, but when you go to take the official test, be prepared, be focused, and do your best the first time!

Secret Key #5 - Test Yourself

Everyone knows that time is money. There is no need to spend too much of your time or too little of your time preparing for the test. You should only spend as much of your precious time preparing as is necessary for you to get the score you need.

Once you have taken a practice test under real conditions of time constraints, then you will know if you are ready for the test or not.

If you have scored extremely high the first time that you take the practice test, then there is not much point in spending countless hours studying. You are already there.

Benchmark your abilities by retaking practice tests and seeing how much you have improved. Once you score high enough to guarantee success, then you are ready.

If you have scored well below where you need, then knuckle down and begin studying in earnest. Check your improvement regularly through the use of practice tests under real conditions. Above all, don't worry, panic, or give up. The key is perseverance!

Then, when you go to take the test, remain confident and remember how well you did on the practice tests. If you can score high enough on a practice test, then you can do the same on the real thing.

General Strategies

The most important thing you can do is to ignore your fears and jump into the test immediately- do not be overwhelmed by any strange-sounding terms. You have to jump into the test like jumping into a pool- all at once is the easiest way.

Make Predictions

As you read and understand the question, try to guess what the answer will be. Remember that several of the answer choices are wrong, and once you begin reading them, your mind will immediately become cluttered with answer choices designed to throw you off. Your mind is typically the most focused immediately after you have read the question and digested its contents. If you can, try to predict what the correct answer will be. You may be surprised at what you can predict.

Quickly scan the choices and see if your prediction is in the listed answer choices. If it is, then you can be quite confident that you have the right answer. It still won't hurt to check the other answer choices, but most of the time, you've got it!

Answer the Question

It may seem obvious to only pick answer choices that answer the question, but the test writers can create some excellent answer choices that are wrong. Don't pick an answer just because it sounds right, or you believe it to be true. It MUST answer the question. Once you've made your selection, always go back and check it against the question and make sure that you didn't misread the question, and the answer choice does answer the question posed.

Benchmark

After you read the first answer choice, decide if you think it sounds correct or not. If it doesn't, move on to the next answer choice. If it does, mentally mark that answer choice. This doesn't mean that you've definitely selected it as your answer choice, it just means that it's the best you've seen thus far. Go ahead and read the next choice. If the next choice is worse than the one you've already selected, keep going to the next answer choice. If the next choice is better than the choice you've already selected, mentally mark the new answer choice as your best guess.

The first answer choice that you select becomes your standard. Every other answer choice must be benchmarked against that standard. That choice is correct until proven otherwise by another answer choice beating it out. Once you've decided that no other answer choice seems as good, do one final check to ensure that your answer choice answers the question posed.

Valid Information

Don't discount any of the information provided in the question. Every piece of information may be necessary to determine the correct answer. None of the information in the question is there to throw you off (while the answer choices will certainly have information to throw you off). If two seemingly unrelated topics are discussed, don't ignore either. You can be confident there is a relationship, or it wouldn't be included in the question, and you are probably going to have to determine what is that relationship to find the answer.

Avoid "Fact Traps"

Don't get distracted by a choice that is factually true. Your search is for the answer that answers the question. Stay focused and don't fall for an answer that is true but incorrect. Always go back to the question and make sure you're choosing an answer that actually answers the question and is not just a true statement. An answer can be factually correct, but it MUST answer the question asked. Additionally, two answers can both be seemingly correct, so be sure to read all of the answer choices, and make sure that you get the one that BEST answers the question.

Milk the Question

Some of the questions may throw you completely off. They might deal with a subject you have not been exposed to, or one that you haven't reviewed in years. While your lack of knowledge about the subject will be a hindrance, the question itself can give you many clues that will help you find the correct answer. Read the question carefully and look for clues. Watch particularly for adjectives and nouns describing difficult terms or words that you don't recognize. Regardless of if you completely understand a word or not, replacing it with a synonym either provided or one you more familiar with may help you to understand what the questions are asking. Rather than wracking your mind about specific detailed information concerning a difficult term or word, try to use mental substitutes that are easier to understand.

The Trap of Familiarity

Don't just choose a word because you recognize it. On difficult questions, you may not recognize a number of words in the answer choices. The test writers don't put "make-believe" words on the test; so don't think that just because you only recognize all the words in one answer choice means that answer choice must be correct. If you only recognize words in one answer choice, then focus on that one. Is it correct? Try your best to determine if it is correct. If it is, that is great, but if it doesn't, eliminate it. Each word and answer choice you eliminate increases your chances of getting the question correct, even if you then have to guess among the unfamiliar choices.

Eliminate Answers

Eliminate choices as soon as you realize they are wrong. But be careful! Make sure you consider all of the possible answer choices. Just because one appears right, doesn't mean that the next one won't be even better! The test writers will usually put more than one good answer choice for every question, so read all of them. Don't worry if you are stuck between two that seem right. By getting down to just two remaining possible choices, your odds are now 50/50. Rather than wasting too much time, play the odds. You are guessing, but guessing wisely, because you've been able to knock out some of the answer choices that you know are wrong. If you are eliminating choices and realize that the last answer choice you are left with is also obviously wrong, don't panic. Start over and consider each choice again. There may easily be something that you missed the first time and will realize on the second pass.

Tough Questions

If you are stumped on a problem or it appears too hard or too difficult, don't waste time. Move on! Remember though, if you can quickly check for obviously incorrect answer choices, your chances of guessing correctly are greatly improved. Before you completely give up, at least try to knock out a couple of possible answers. Eliminate what you can and then guess at the remaining answer choices before moving on.

Brainstorm

If you get stuck on a difficult question, spend a few seconds quickly brainstorming. Run through the complete list of possible answer choices. Look at each choice and ask yourself, "Could this answer the question satisfactorily?" Go through each answer choice and consider it independently of the other. By systematically going through all possibilities, you may find something that you would otherwise overlook. Remember that when you get stuck, it's important to try to keep moving.

Read Carefully

Understand the problem. Read the question and answer choices carefully. Don't miss the question because you misread the terms. You have plenty of time to read each question thoroughly and make sure you understand what is being asked. Yet a happy medium must be attained, so don't waste too much time. You must read carefully, but efficiently.

Face Value

When in doubt, use common sense. Always accept the situation in the problem at face value. Don't read too much into it. These problems will not require you to make huge leaps of logic. The test writers aren't trying to throw you off with a cheap trick. If you have to go beyond creativity and make a leap of logic in order to have an answer choice answer the question, then you should look at the other answer choices. Don't overcomplicate the problem by creating theoretical relationships or explanations that will warp time or space. These are normal problems rooted in reality. It's just that the applicable relationship or explanation may not be readily apparent and you have to figure things out. Use your common sense to interpret anything that isn't clear.

Prefixes

If you're having trouble with a word in the question or answer choices, try dissecting it. Take advantage of every clue that the word might include. Prefixes and suffixes can be a huge help. Usually they allow you to determine a basic meaning. Pre- means before, post- means after, pro - is positive, de- is negative. From these prefixes and suffixes, you can get an idea of the general meaning of the word and try to put it into context. Beware though of any traps. Just because con is the opposite of pro, doesn't necessarily mean congress is the opposite of progress!

Hedge Phrases

Watch out for critical "hedge" phrases, such as likely, may, can, will often, sometimes, often, almost, mostly, usually, generally, rarely, sometimes. Question writers insert these hedge phrases to cover every possibility. Often an answer choice will be wrong simply because it leaves no room for exception. Avoid answer choices that have definitive words like "exactly," and "always".

Switchback Words

Stay alert for "switchbacks". These are the words and phrases frequently used to alert you to shifts in thought. The most common switchback word is "but". Others include although, however, nevertheless, on the other hand, even though, while, in spite of, despite, regardless of.

New Information

Correct answer choices will rarely have completely new information included. Answer choices typically are straightforward reflections of the material asked about and will directly relate to the question. If a new piece of information is included in an answer choice that doesn't even seem to relate to the topic being asked about, then that answer choice is likely incorrect. All of the information needed to answer the question is usually provided for you, and so you should not have to make guesses that are unsupported or choose answer choices that require unknown information that cannot be reasoned on its own.

Time Management

On technical questions, don't get lost on the technical terms. Don't spend too much time on any one question. If you don't know what a term means, then since you don't have a dictionary, odds are you aren't going to get much further. You should immediately recognize terms as whether or not you know them. If you don't, work with the other clues that you have, the other answer choices and terms provided, but don't waste too much time trying to figure out a difficult term.

Contextual Clues

Look for contextual clues. An answer can be right but not correct. The contextual clues will help you find the answer that is most right and is correct. Understand the context in which a phrase or statement is made. This will help you make important distinctions.

Don't Panic

Panicking will not answer any questions for you. Therefore, it isn't helpful. When you first see the question, if your mind goes blank, take a deep breath. Force yourself to mechanically go through the steps of solving the problem and using the strategies you've learned.

Pace Yourself

Don't get clock fever. It's easy to be overwhelmed when you're looking at a page full of questions, your mind is full of random thoughts and feeling confused, and the clock is ticking down faster than you would like. Calm down and maintain the pace that you have set for yourself. As long as you are on track by monitoring your pace, you are guaranteed to have enough time for yourself. When you get to the last few minutes of the test, it may seem like you won't have enough time left, but if you only have as many questions as you should have left at that point, then you're right on track!

Answer Selection

The best way to pick an answer choice is to eliminate all of those that are wrong, until only one is left and confirm that is the correct answer. Sometimes though, an answer choice may immediately look right. Be careful! Take a second to make sure that the other choices are not equally obvious. Don't make a hasty mistake. There are only two times that you should stop before checking other answers. First is when you are positive that the answer choice you have selected is correct. Second is when time is almost out and you have to make a quick guess!

Check Your Work

Since you will probably not know every term listed and the answer to every question, it is important that you get credit for the ones that you do know. Don't miss any questions through careless mistakes. If at all possible, try to take a second to look back over your answer selection and make sure you've selected the correct answer choice and haven't made a costly careless mistake (such as marking an answer choice that you didn't mean to mark). This quick double check should more than pay for itself in caught mistakes for the time it costs.

Beware of Directly Quoted Answers

Sometimes an answer choice will repeat word for word a portion of the question or reference section. However, beware of such exact duplication – it may be a trap! More than likely, the correct choice will paraphrase or summarize a point, rather than being exactly the same wording.

Slang

Scientific sounding answers are better than slang ones. An answer choice that begins "To compare the outcomes…" is much more likely to be correct than one that begins "Because some people insisted…"

Extreme Statements

Avoid wild answers that throw out highly controversial ideas that are proclaimed as established fact. An answer choice that states the "process should be used in certain situations, if…" is much more likely to be correct than one that states the "process should be discontinued completely." The first is a calm rational statement and doesn't even make a definitive, uncompromising stance, using a hedge word "if" to provide wiggle room, whereas the second choice is a radical idea and far more extreme.

Answer Choice Families

When you have two or more answer choices that are direct opposites or parallels, one of them is usually the correct answer. For instance, if one answer choice states "x increases" and another answer choice states "x decreases" or "y increases," then those two or three answer choices are very similar in construction and fall into the same family of answer choices. A family of answer choices is when two or three answer choices are very similar in construction, and yet often have a directly opposite meaning. Usually the correct answer choice will be in that family of answer choices. The "odd man out" or answer choice that doesn't seem to fit the parallel construction of the other answer choices is more likely to be incorrect.

Be Aware of the Following:

1. 150 questions are given on the EMT-P test.
2. Questions are not divided into nice categories. They are completely random.
3. Questions can ask content or be based on a mini-case.
4. Make sure you know your CPR backwards and forwards before taking the exam.
5. Review all of the information in this manual.